Towards Better Reproductive
Health
in Eastern Europe

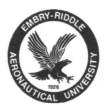

Towards Better Reproductive Health
in Eastern Europe

Concern, Commitment, and Change

Edited by

G. LINDMARK, M. HORGA, A. CAMPANA,
and J. KASONDE

WHO Scientific Working Group on Reproductive Health Research

⁖CEUPRESS

Central European
University Press

World Health
Organization

Published by

Central European University Press
Október 6. utca 12
H-1051 Budapest
Hungary

400 West 59th Street
New York, NY 10019
USA

Distributed by
Plymbridge Distributors Ltd., Estover Road, Plymouth PL6 7PZ,
United Kingdom

ISBN 963-9116-30-0

Graphic artwork on cover by Tamás Karácsony and Tamás Maros

Library of Congress Cataloging in Publication Data
A CIP catalog record for this book is available upon request

Printed in Hungary by Akadémiai Nyomda Kft.

Contents

v

List of tables

List of figures

List of contributors

- I. Auzina, Medical Academy of Latvia, Riga, Latvia
- G. Benagiano, WHO, Geneva, Switzerland
- A. Brandrup-Lukanow, WHO Regional Office for Europe, Sexual and Family Health Unit, Copenhagen, Denmark
- A. Campana, University Hospital, Geneva, Switzerland
- A. Gromyko, WHO Regional Office for Europe, Copenhagen, Denmark
- H. Honkanen, WHO, Geneva, Switzerland
- M. Horga, Center of Public Health, Targu-Mures, Romania
- L. Kovács, Albert Szent-Györgyi Medical University, Szeged, Hungary
- G. Lazdane, Medical Academy of Latvia, Riga, Latvia
- G. Lindmark, University Hospital, Uppsala, Sweden
- F. Lüdicke, University Hospital, Geneva, Switzerland

Foreword

In the field of international health the twentieth century will go down in history as the period of the greatest advances in health technology and health care; and in these achievements Europe will be known to have played a leading role. But the discrepancies in health and health care status between the market economies of the West and the transitional economies of the East have shown a glaring gap, especially in the last decade of the century. This gap has been particularly prominent in the area of reproductive health.

The scientific community in both the East and the West has fortunately risen to the challenge. The development of technologies and the generation of knowledge have proceeded faster than ever, providing policymakers with the tools they need to respond to the challenge. Programs and services that had degenerated in difficult economic circumstances have begun to improve tremendously, justifying the hope that the status of health and health care in the whole region will attain even higher levels in coming years.

The WHO Region of Europe has shown leadership in the movement to improve health in general and reproductive health in particular. Policymakers and program managers in the member states of the Region now have an added tool in the information provided in these pages. Let them use this knowledge to achieve better reproductive health in Eastern Europe. I urge them to take up the challenge.

J. E. Asvall

Regional Director
WHO Regional Office for Europe

Reproductive health in Eastern Europe: an overview and the challenges ahead

HELENA HONKANEN and GIUSEPPE BENAGIANO

UNDP/UNFPA/WHO/World Bank Special Programme of Research, Development and Research Training in Human Reproduction, Geneva, Switzerland

Abstract

The countries of Eastern Europe are in transition not only economically but also culturally. Reproductive health indicators show that the prevalence of contraceptive use is low, abortion rates are high, maternal and infant mortality are rising, and the incidence of sexually transmitted diseases shows an upward trend. As the political climate changed in Eastern Europe, more opportunities arose to promote cooperation between research centers in Eastern and Western Europe. To facilitate this cooperation, the Special Programme of Research, Development and Research Training in Human Reproduction recently established a Scientific Working Group on Reproductive Health Research in Eastern Europe to coordinate research and research training activities in the region.

To improve reproductive health in Eastern Europe, health care delivery also needs to be improved; to achieve this, training of health care personnel is required to allow them to obtain updated information; education, especially for adolescents, on sexual and contraceptive matters is at the center of the new agenda; and more research is needed on reproductive health in general.

1

Introduction

For the purpose of WHO activities in this region, Eastern Europe covers the Baltic states, the countries of Central and Eastern Europe, the Commonwealth of Independent States, the former Soviet Central Asian Republics and Kazakhstan, and the countries of former Yugoslavia. A list of these countries is provided as an Appendix.

This huge area is by no means uniform. A woman in Turkmenistan has a life expectancy of 62 years, a man 69 years. A Russian woman can expect to live 72 years, a man only 59 years. As a comparison, in Western Europe life expectancy varies between 70 years for a man and 78 years for a woman in Portugal, and 75 years for a man and 81 years for a woman in Switzerland (Monnier, and De Guibert-Lantoine, 1995).

In Russia the mean number of livebirths per woman is 1.4, close to that of most Western European countries, where the birthrate is usually under 2. In the Central Asian Republics, on the other hand, the total fertility rate is much higher: in Tajikistan it is 5.0 and in Turkmenistan 4.1 (Monnier, and De Guibert-Lantoine, 1995).

Characteristics of reproductive health in Eastern Europe

Contraceptive prevalence is low

The overall utilization of modern methods of contraception in the region is usually low. Prevalence varies from 7% in Azerbaijan to 60% in Hungary (fig. 1.1). Intrauterine devices are the most widely used methods in Russia, the Central Asian Republics, and the Baltic states (80% of users of modern methods), whereas in Hungary the most popular method is the oral contraceptive pill (WHO and UN Population Fund, 1995).

The reasons for not using effective methods and for the preference for certain methods vary from country to country. Also, the availability of contraceptives has varied. For instance, in 1966, concerned about the low rate of population growth, the Romanian government prohibited not only abortion but also sex education and contraception, and imposed a ban on the sale and the importation of contraceptives (United Nations, 1995). After the revolution in December 1989, abortion was legalized again, and the restrictions on the importation and sale of contraceptives were removed. However, because of this long gap, the use of modern methods is fairly low—about 14% (IOMC and CDC, 1995).

In many countries there is simply a lack of effective contraceptives. But even in countries where contraceptives are theoretically available, there are obstacles to widespread utilization. If contraceptives are not produced within the country, they have to be imported and paid for with hard currency, which makes them unaffordable for many people.

Besides availability and affordability, other obstacles prevent widespread use. First and foremost is a lack of knowledge about contraceptives, both among the population and among providers. There are also misconceptions about the safety of modern contraceptives. For example, in Russia and Romania many women believe that oral contraceptives are harmful to their health and should not be used (IOMC and CDC, 1995). For this reason, more research concerning sexual behavior and the knowledge, attitudes, and practice of contraception is needed in order to change the situation. Also, proper training for providers and educational programs for consumers are badly needed.

To better evaluate the situation, the Special Programme recently launched a multicenter study on what determines the choice and use of methods of fertility regulation in Eastern Europe. The objectives of this study are: to assess the characteristics of women

3

who come to participating institutions seeking an abortion but do not use modern methods of contraception, and compare them to users of modern methods; to determine the perceptions and factors that influence the acceptance or refusal of contraception; and to identify possible problems encountered with service providers. This is one of the studies developed by the Scientific Working Group on Reproductive Health Research in Eastern Europe (SWG).

Sex education in schools is nonexistent in most Eastern European countries; thus there is an urgent need to introduce both sex education and education about contraception into the school curriculum, because adolescence is the time when people should be encouraged to establish safe and responsible patterns of sexual behavior for the rest of their lives.

Abortion rates are still high

Most countries in Eastern Europe have a very high prevalence of induced abortion. The historical reason for this is the nonavailability of contraceptive methods; even where some could be obtained, there has been no real knowledge about them and abortion has been, for all practical purposes, the most important method of fertility regulation. In Hungary the abortion rate is 33/1000 women per year aged 15–44 years, in the Russian Federation it is 82/1000, but the highest rate is found in Romania at 140/1000. For comparison, in Western Europe France has a rate of 13/1000 and Finland 8 /1000 (fig. 1.2).

Another way to look at abortion statistics is to compare them with birthrates. In 1993 in the Russian Federation, as many as 214 abortions per 100 births were performed. Again there are regional differences. In the Baltic states the rate is somewhat lower; for example, in Latvia in 1994 it was 129 per 100 births. The lowest rate is found in the Central Asian Republics, where in 1994 it was 88 per 100 births in Kazakhstan (fig. 1.3).

4

As mentioned above, prior to 1989 the Romanian government held strong pronatalist views; contraception was banned and abortion was illegal. After the 1989 revolution, when abortion was legalized and safe abortion made available, the reality of abortion being used as a method of birth control surfaced again. Abortion rates in Romania are the highest in the world: in 1992 there were 270 abortions per 100 births, most of them performed among married women who have achieved the desired family size (IOMC and CDC, 1995).

In Poland in 1993 Parliament approved a law which permits abortion only when the pregnancy threatens the life or health of the mother, when the fetus has a serious malformation, or in cases of rape or incest. This led to a surge in illegal abortions and in women traveling to neighboring countries for abortion. Because of this, in 1996 the abortion law was relaxed again.

These facts underline an important concept: in most countries a law that forbids abortion does not really result in a decrease in the number of women who resort to the procedure to stop an unwanted pregnancy. The problem is that illegal abortions are often unsafe and the consequences can be seen in the increased morbidity related to pregnancy, in higher rates of secondary infertility, and in the mortality among pregnant women. Romania is a perfect example of this: banning abortion resulted in the highest maternal mortality in Europe, with 85% of deaths related to pregnancy attributable to unsafe abortions. In 1989 there were 159 maternal deaths per 100 000 livebirths; the next year, after abortion was legalized and the procedure became much safer, mortality during pregnancy or delivery fell to 83 per 100 000 livebirths (IOMC and CDC, 1995).

To move successfully from abortion to contraception, people's attitudes and behavior must be changed. This requires massive training and education programs, as well as the will of the government. For example, in Estonia, where abortion is legal, the government has adopted a policy whereby women are charged for abortion services and this money is then used to subsidize contraceptives.

Maternal mortality is high

Morbidity and mortality related to pregnancy are relatively high in Eastern Europe and because abortion is so widely used as a method of regulating fertility, it remains a major cause of maternal mortality in many countries of the region. Poor socioeconomic conditions and limited access to safe and effective health services are other causes of this phenomenon. Compared with Western Europe, where maternal mortality is below 10 per 100 000 births, in 1992 in Tajikistan there were 83 maternal deaths per 100 000 livebirths (fig. 1.4). The main causes of death were bleeding and toxemia (WHO, 1995).

Sexually transmitted diseases (STDs) show a rising trend

During the 1990s in Eastern Europe there was a rapid increase in the incidence of STDs. For instance, in the Russian Federation between 1989 and 1995, probably as a consequence of major social changes and of the disruption of existing health services, there was a fortyfold increase in the incidence of syphilis (WHO Regional Office for Europe, unpublished data). These figures are worrying because the spread of STDs has many important negative effects, like pelvic inflammatory disease, which can cause tubal blockage and lead to infertility, ectopic pregnancies, and chronic pain. In addition, the human papillomavirus and chlamydia are important risk factors for cervical cancer.

6

To monitor the spread of STDs, a unified system of data collection needs to be introduced. At present, in many Eastern European countries only some STDs (such as the human immunodeficiency virus, hepatitis B virus, syphilis, and gonorrhea) have to be reported, whereas others like chlamydia do not. The AIDS epidemic seems to have reached Eastern Europe six to seven years later than Western Europe, but the number of HIV-positive people is rising.

An important factor in the spread of STDs is the major change in people's lives brought about by the transition from socialist to market economies. People are allowed to travel abroad and there are more tourists coming to visit these formerly closed countries. Unfortunately, so-called "sex tourism" also flourishes, because in many countries high unemployment has forced a growing number of people to earn their living by prostitution.

Infant mortality is high

Infant mortality in Eastern European countries far exceeds that in Western Europe. The lowest rate in Eastern Europe is 8 per 1000 livebirths in the Czech Republic; in the Russian Federation it is 18 per 1000 and in the Central Asian Republics it is even higher, for example, 53 in Turkmenistan (fig. 1.5). This compares with an average in the European Union of 8 per 1000 livebirths. An SWG research project was started in 1996 in various Eastern European countries to investigate the reasons for perinatal deaths.

The work of the Special Programme

The Special Programme of Research, Development and Research Training in Human Reproduction (HRP) is cosponsored by the United Nations Development Program (UNDP), the United Nations Population Fund (UNFPA), the World Health Organization

(WHO), and the World Bank, and it is the main group within the United Nations carrying out reproductive health research.

The Programme's priorities include research on: new methods of fertility regulation for both women and men; the introduction of such methods into family planning programs; the long-term safety of methods already in use; social and behavioral aspects of reproductive health, and methods of controlling the spread of STDs, which can cause infertility. The Programme also carries out activities to strengthen the research capabilities of developing countries to enable them to meet their own research needs and participate in the global effort in reproductive health research (WHO, 1996).

History of the East European initiative

As the political climate changed in Eastern Europe, better opportunities arose to promote scientific cooperation between centers in Eastern and Western Europe. An East–West European Initiative for Research on Reproductive Health was launched in 1990 during a meeting in Szeged, Hungary, with the support of HRP. The objectives of this initiative were to exchange information in the field of reproduction; to assess common research needs and priorities in reproductive health; to develop collaborative plans between centers; and to explore ways to mobilize resources for research (WHO, 1991).

A second meeting was held in Szeged in 1993 to assess the research and service needs in reproductive health in Eastern Europe and to propose ways and means to improve—through collaboration—the reproductive health status of the populations of these countries. The main problems identified were the lack of common definitions and adequate statistical data; the lack of training of professionals; deficiencies in knowledge about current family planning methods among professionals, consumers, policymakers, and media representatives; lack of supplies of modern

8

contraceptives; lack of sex education in schools; high levels of maternal mortality, induced abortions, and infertility; and inability to prevent, diagnose, and treat STDs. The summary and the recommendations of the meeting were published in a document called The Szeged Declaration (1994).

The SWG

The SWG on Reproductive Health Research in Eastern Europe was established with the help and support of HRP to coordinate research and research training activities and to advise on the allocation of funds. At the time this paper was written, the SWG comprised members from Armenia, the Czech Republic, Hungary, Romania, Sweden, and Switzerland. It organizes an annual meeting that is attended by representatives from Eastern European countries, by the WHO Secretariat, and by advisers and observers from various organizations with an interest in reproductive health in Eastern Europe.

The SWG first met in May 1994, developed research projects involving centers in Eastern Europe, and drew up a program for research training. Projects approved so far address three major areas of reproductive health: fertility regulation, perinatal care, and the health consequences of induced abortion. All projects are multinational, which allows these topics to be studied simultaneously in several Eastern European countries. This multinational approach is also expected to strengthen collaboration among participating countries. The results of the research will be brought to the attention of people at policy- and decision-making level in order to improve services.

The challenge

Because the countries of Eastern Europe are in a transitional phase, not only economically but also culturally, it is a great challenge to improve their reproductive health status. In most of these countries, there are adequate numbers of trained personnel and a number of well-established scientific institutions which could have the potential, if they receive help from outside, to address and solve the problems associated with reproduction.

It is generally agreed that, to improve the reproductive health status of the people of Eastern European countries, the following actions are needed:

a. an improvement in health care delivery;

b. the provision of proper information for the public, for example, on different family planning methods;

c. the provision of adequate training for health personnel, including updated information;

d. the provision of modern education for all age groups, but especially for adolescents—sex and contraceptive education should be introduced into the school curriculum;

e. more research on aspects of reproductive health that are specific to these countries.

Policymakers should be made aware that research is one of the most cost-effective means of solving problems, including those of reproductive health.

Conclusions

This brief overview of the status of reproductive health in Eastern Europe shows clearly that the task ahead is monumental. There is an urgent need for scientists to evaluate and monitor developments and to provide policymakers with correct, updated information to design effective reproductive health care programs. It is right and proper that the International Federation of Gynecology and Obstetrics should focus on the problems of this subregion. Together we must take the necessary actions to improve reproductive health in Central and Eastern Europe.

References

IOMC and CDC. 1995. *Reproductive health survey, Romania, 1993.* Bucharest: Institute for Mother and Child Care & Division of Reproductive Health, Centers for Disease Control and Prevention.

Monnier, A., and De Guibert-Lantoine, C. 1995. The demographic situation of Europe and the developed countries overseas: an annual report. *Population, an English Selection* 7:187–202.

WHO. 1991. Special Programme of Research, Development and Research Training in Human Reproduction. 1991. *East–West European initiative for research on reproductive health.* Geneva: World Health Organization.

WHO. 1996. Special Programme of Research, Development and Research Training in Human Reproduction. 1996. *Biennial report 1994–1995.* Geneva: World Health Organization.

The Szeged Declaration. 1994. Assessment of research and service needs on reproductive health in Eastern Europe—concerns and commitment. *Human Reproduction* 9: 750–2.

United Nations. 1992. *Abortion policies: a global review.* New York: United Nations.

United Nations. 1995. *Abortion policies: a global review,* Volume III, pp. 52–53. New York: United Nations, Department for Economic and Social Information and Policy Analysis, Population Division.

WHO Regional Office for Europe. 1995. *Highlights on women's health in Europe.* Doc: EUR/ICP/FMLY 94 01/PB02. Copenhagen: World Health Organization.

WHO Regional Office for Europe and United Nations Population Fund. 1995. Family planning and reproductive health in CCEE/NIS. Doc. EUR/ICP/FMLY 94 03/PB01. Copenhagen: World Health Organization.

Appendix

List of countries

The Baltic states

Estonia

Latvia

Lithuania

Central and Eastern Europe

Albania

Bulgaria

Czech Republic

Hungary

Poland

Romania

Slovakia

Commonwealth of Independent States

Armenia

Azerbaijan

Belarus

Georgia

Republic of Moldova

Russian Federation

Ukraine

Central Asian Republics and Kazakhstan

Kazakhstan

Kyrgyzstan

Tajikistan

Turkmenistan

Uzbekistan

Former Yugoslavia

Bosnia and Herzegovina

Croatia

Slovenia

The Former Yugoslav
Republic of Macedonia

Yugoslavia

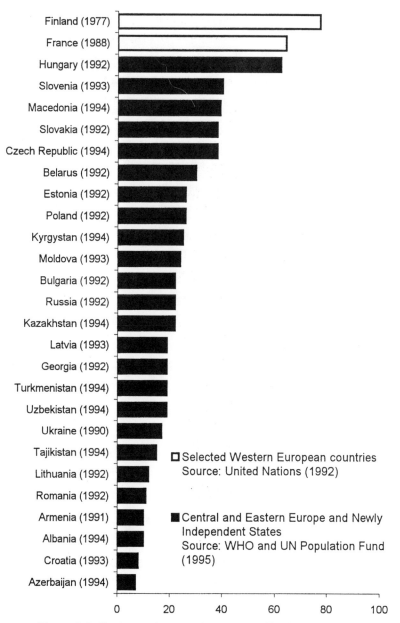

Figure 1.1. Contraceptive prevalence rate (effective methods)
for 100 married women.

13

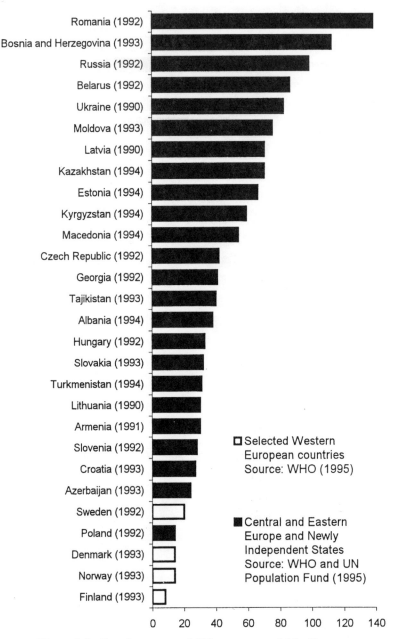

Figure 1.2. Abortion rate per 1000 women aged 15–49 years.

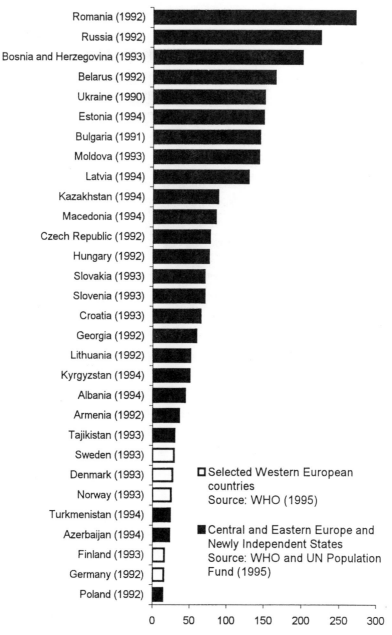

Figure 1.3. Abortion to birth ratio per 100 births.

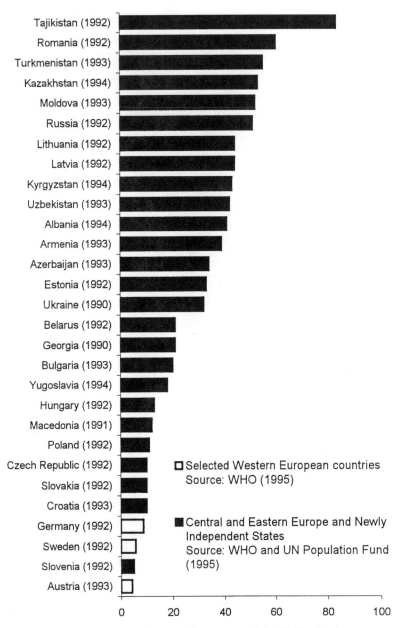

Figure 1.4. Maternal mortality rate per 100 000 live births.

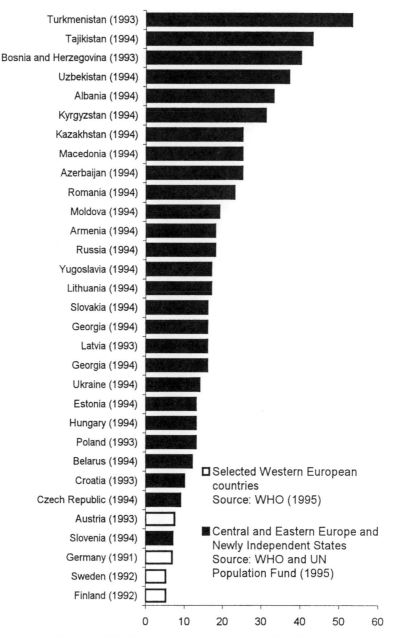

Figure 1.5. Infant mortality rate per 1000 live births.

17

Can a process of quality assurance improve pregnancy outcome?

GUNILLA LINDMARK

Department of Obstetrics and Gynecology,
University of Uppsala, Uppsala, Sweden

Abstract

Pregnancy outcome for mothers and infants in terms of complication rates and survival are considered to be key indicators of the health status and of the health services available to any given population. These indicators are particularly sensitive to differences and changes in socioeconomic standards and national welfare programs. It is therefore of great concern that countries in Eastern Europe have figures for maternal and perinatal mortality considerably higher than those of other industrialized countries—in fact often on level with or higher than figures from medium income developing countries. Recent statistics even suggest an increase in mortality figures in some countries or subgroups of the population. In the report of WHO and UN Population Fund from 1995, none of the countries in the former Soviet Union report a maternal mortality below the EURO target of 15 per 100 000 (fig. 2.1). In this report, perinatal mortality is not reported, but infant mortality rates of 30–50 per 1000 livebirths are reported from several countries, and only two, the Czech Republic and Slovenia, have infant mortality rates below 10, which is the European target (fig. 2.2). Since neonatal mortality is usually two thirds of infant mortality, this will of course also affect perinatal mortality. In the most recent statistics published by the WHO Safe

19

Motherhood Program (WHO/FRH/MSM/96.7), perinatal mortality rates from Eastern Europe and the Baltic states are two to three times higher than in Northern and Western Europe. As a consequence of the dramatic social and economic changes in many of these countries in transition, there is a risk that this difference will increase. At the same time, resources for and access to health care may decrease. In such a situation, the quality of the health care given is of vital importance for its impact on the total maternal and perinatal health situation.

Quality assurance in maternal health care

It is becoming increasingly clear that the delivery of health care services should not be discussed only in quantitative terms, which is still often the case, but also in terms of quality. In a situation where there are considerable health problems and limited access to services, health care is often described quantitatively in number of contacts or procedures performed, but the qualitative dimensions of health care are fundamental if it is to make a difference to the health of people. This is emphasized by increasing demands from clients—not least in maternal health care—to be considered as individuals and not only as objectives of health care activities. Since even in the most affluent parts of the world resources are restricted and do not permit unlimited health care interventions, the demand for critical scrutiny and assessment of the quality of health care is also increasing (Meeker, 1994).

Quality in health care, as in other client-oriented activities, can be defined as the "ability to meet the needs" of the users of the services (Deming, 1986). In maternal and perinatal health care, the best possible outcome of pregnancy is naturally a priority. However, even though survival of mother and baby without short-term or long-term morbidity is the foremost requirement, there are other needs related to social, cultural, and existential dimensions that also have to be considered in the care of mothers and infants. It is important in any health care system that these dimensions are acknowledged or the acceptance of and compliance with care will otherwise decrease.

The health care system alone cannot meet the medical and broader health needs related to pregnancy. Pregnancy outcome is related to the standard of health care and access to it; it is also related to general living standards, including education, working conditions, housing and hygiene, lifestyle, and cultural and social circumstances. It is therefore appropriate that pregnancy outcome variables as well as other indicators of reproductive health are considered as important indicators of overall living conditions in a society or in a subgroup of a population. Although the relative importance for health of health care interventions in relation to other factors is debatable, it is the responsibility of health care workers to do their utmost to meet the patient's expectations of the best possible outcome. To maintain and improve quality in health care, it is necessary to define clearly the goals and objectives related to patients' needs and to assess available resources (Loegering, Reiter, and Gambone, 1994). The process of quality assurance is defined as a planned and systematic critical analysis of the quality of care (International Quality Standards, ISO 9000). Such an analysis includes the procedures used for diagnosis and treatment, the use of resources, and the outcomes and quality of life for women and their babies. In order to achieve an improvement in quality, this assessment must be built into an ongoing process, whereby results are continuously fed back and discussed with all those involved at all levels of the health care system (fig. 2.3).

Another term for this process is continuous quality improvement (Deming, 1986). It is emphasized that, for appropriate delivery of care, it is essential to have practice guidelines that define the content of care and the management of patient problems (Meeker, 1994). Monitoring of care can be performed through clinical in-

21

dicators that show important aspects of care that can be measured or counted, that identify needs, and that can be used to monitor progress. When quality of care is evaluated, these indicators are assessed with the peer review criteria of appropriateness, process, outcome, and cost-effectiveness.

Quality indicators in maternal health care

A model often used for analysis of quality addresses three aspects of quality (Donabedian, 1978): indicators of quality can be applied to (1) the structure of health care, (2) its organization, and (3) available resources. Quality indicators can also be defined that relate to the process or utilization of these resources in the provision of health care. Such indicators can assess the extent to which each activity carried out for screening, prevention, diagnosis, or therapy is correctly applied or is being used for the purpose for which it is intended or appropriate.

Quality assessment of the structure of care addresses the resources including staff qualifications and structured and adequate programs of care. In maternal health care, the structured patient file is of special importance for quality and is intermittently linked to the content and direction of the care given.

Assessment of the quality of the process includes ascertaining if care is carried out according to the plan, guidelines, or recommendations. It should also include a critical assessment of the appropriateness of these components. The best and ultimate quality indicator should of course relate to the result of the health care process in terms of mortality, morbidity, patient satisfaction, or level of knowledge.

Mortality figures are often reported and used as result indicators (Shaw, 1990). Maternal and neonatal morbidity are not as clear-cut and are subject to considerable variation in definition. It is rare

22

that mothers or infants are examined systematically to record morbidity indicators. Proxy indicators are therefore often used, such as a prolonged stay in hospital, transfer for other forms of care, or use of neonatal intensive care. The difficulties in neonatal quality control compared with the assessment of quality in obstetric care have been pointed out (Jahrig, Jahrig, and Heinrich, 1988). For infants, the health outcomes of great importance relate to later development and handicaps that can only be detected by long-term follow-up, a resource-demanding procedure with considerable methodological difficulties (Gaffney et al., 1994). Another problem is that long-term morbidity that may result from health care interventions cannot be immediately assessed and will be difficult to distinguish from other influences.

Even if mortality and morbidity are important quality indicators, they are most suitable for comparisons at a regional, national, or international level. Due to natural and random variation and relatively low absolute figures, they are less useful for quality assurance in individual clinics or health care units. It also must be taken into account that perinatal and maternal mortality and morbidity are endpoints in a long chain of events so that it can be difficult to estimate the relative importance of each on the final outcome. Maternal and perinatal care consists of a number of screening systems combined with planned as well as emergency interventions, all of which are conducted by several successive groups of health care workers in different settings.

Outcome variables such as maternal satisfaction, ability to breast feed and level of relevant knowledge can be assessed and related more directly to the quality of specific parts of the health care program. Assessment of different aspects of midwifery care is increasingly used for quality assurance (Wiegers et al., 1996).

Clinical quality indicators useful for monitoring results have been developed. One example is the list by the American College of Obstetricians and Gynecologists (table 2.1). This list focuses

23

on severe complications and the need for medical interventions that are directly related to management decisions, which are known to vary considerably among clinicians and institutions. The list also includes events such as delivery of a premature infant in an institution without appropriate resources. Such indicators clearly will be relevant only in situations where a well-defined guideline for the overall organization of care exists.

Still another approach to recording outcome indicators is to concentrate on those that are considered to be influenced by the process of care and its quality (Buekens, 1990). In addition to maternal and perinatal mortality, postpartum hemorrhage, sequelae of obstructed labor, Apgar score, and very early neonatal seizures have been suggested.

Another example of a list of essential quality indicators for maternal and perinatal care is given by the European Consensus Conference of Quality Indicators for Perinatal Care, a project coordinated by WHO/EURO/IMI (table 2.2). These indicators were developed in a consensus discussion by 53 experts from 24 European countries and tested at local, regional, and national levels. The indicators were chosen for relevance and feasibility, including the possibility of defining and recording them.

European variation in quality indicators

When the quality indicators were compared among countries, it could be clearly demonstrated that profound differences exist between the majority of the European Union countries and countries in Eastern Europe. The differences are sometimes dramatic, as for eclampsia, where there is an average of 203 cases per 100 000 deliveries in the Newly Independent States of the former Soviet Union (NIS) compared with an average of 29 per 100 000 for Western European countries (fig. 2.4). However, it can also be seen from figure 2.4 that the variation between the countries in the

NIS is as large as between the groups of countries. An example of process-related indicators is the proportion of women in labor receiving blood transfusions (fig. 2.5). Here the variation between institutions is even larger than between groups of countries, reflecting not only differences in resources, such as access to the drug oxytocin and skilled obstetric interventions, but also the lack of a clear understanding of appropriate indications for blood transfusion, which is a rather powerful intervention.

The variation in intrapartum deaths (fig. 2.6) can be discussed together with the corresponding variation in the rates for cesarean section (fig. 2.7). Although it may seem that similar patterns exist between rates for cesarean sections, with an inverse correlation to poor pregnancy outcomes, it must be emphasized that cesarean rates above 6–10% show no positive correlation with improved maternal and fetal outcome.

These examples demonstrate the usefulness of such quality indicators for constructive discussions about the content and quality of maternal health care. It is also clear that the variations in outcome cannot be related to physical resources in a simple way, but again must be discussed in the wider context of the attitudes, practices, and knowledge of health staff at all levels.

In the assessment of the results of care, it is always a danger that the assessment is limited to intermediate variables such as results of tests or examinations, and not to direct patient-related measures of quality of life. Also, in perinatal care it is not uncommon that, as the gold standard for a screening procedure or an intervention during pregnancy, the result of another test or examination is used and not a parameter directly related to the actual health outcome of mother of infant. This is not to say that variables that are indirectly related to health outcome cannot be used. It is often appropriate to use a variable such as low birthweight as a morbidity outcome, since it has a direct relation to short- and long-term morbidity in the infant.

Data collection for monitoring quality

Various methods can be used to collect data for quality assurance. Whenever possible, existing data that has been routinely collected should be used in order to limit the use of more resources (Hall, 1993). Local statistics of pregnancy outcome and health care activities are the basis for all kinds of assessment of structure as well as process. Most health care institutions have such statistics, but for comparisons, not only of trends over time in a specific institution, but also between institutions or using the data compiled for nationwide comparisons, it is essential that all variables are defined according to international standards. Even the definition of basic concepts like perinatal mortality is not uniform in all centers, and in many centers in Eastern Europe birthweights less than 1000 g or gestational ages less than 28 weeks are not included in the statistics. It is also common in several Eastern European countries that only low-birthweight infants who survive the first week are reported. It is of great importance for perinatal outcome for the lowest birthweight classes to be included. Data from Estonia demonstrate the differences in perinatal mortality if the 500 g cutoff is used (table 2.3).

When it comes to cause of death, even more problematic are local registers, diagnosis of complications, and autopsy data. Terms such as hypoxia, placental dysfunction, or pre-eclampsia are frequently used without clear and uniform definitions of the variables. It is therefore doubtful if autopsy data really are as helpful for quality studies as has been claimed (Hagerstrand, and Lundberg, 1993; Cartlidge et al., 1995). Important routine data collection systems that give the denominators for statistics are civil registration of births and deaths and clinical information systems in hospitals or primary care centers. In many countries routine surveys that cover aspects of reproductive health are repeated at regular intervals. When general child health care services are functioning, data from such follow-up visits can also be used to

26

describe morbidity. Centralized case-based birth registers are still not prevalent in Eastern Europe, but are important means of monitoring maternal and perinatal health.

The patient chart is another important quality instrument if it is standardized and contains specified and well defined data. Computerization can simplify the production of statistics (Sokol, Chik, and Zador, 1992). Special standards for records in obstetrics and gynecology have been published (Maresh, and Hall, 1991). It has to be emphasized that unless there are specific requirements for registration of a certain variable, it is unlikely that it is useful for quality assessment—for example, maternal symptoms or events that are subject to individual judgment (Jahn, and Berle, 1996; Hutchon, 1996). In general, all data that are filtered through a process of subjective interpretation are less reliable than absolute values and test results.

Specific surveys and interviews as well as observations of the process of care are valuable instruments for assessment of quality, but they cannot usually be routinely used since they are resource-demanding and also depend on the training and skills of the performer. They therefore have to be limited to specific questions during short periods.

Classifying and auditing perinatal deaths

An important instrument for quality assessment on a case-basis is perinatal audit (Dunn, and McIlwaine, 1996). An audit can be structured so that the specific level of care at which action should be taken can be defined. One such model for audit has been developed in the Scandinavian countries. It was first used in a Danish–Swedish study (Langhoff-Roos et al., 1996), but has now been extended to the Baltic states and the Russian Federation. This audit classification of perinatal deaths takes into account the following variables:

1. Fetal malformations.

2. Time of death in relation to delivery (before admission, between admission and birth, and after birth in the early neonatal period).

3. Significant growth retardation (operationalized as a baby born small for gestational age with birthweight below a mean of –2 standard deviations).

4. Gestational age in completed weeks (less than 28 weeks, 28–33 weeks, and above 34 weeks in neonatal deaths).

5. Apgar score less than 7 at 5 minutes (in neonatal deaths).

These variables can be used to form 12 categories of perinatal death that have proven very useful as a practical means of comparing perinatal outcome on a national basis and indicating areas of concern (table 2.4).

It is possible to define the five basic variables clearly and they are usually routinely recorded. Fetal malformation is the only one open to subjective judgment, but, usually, gross malformation that could cause fetal or neonatal death is less open to misclassification than more minor malformations. Each of these five groups can be discussed in terms of potential avoidance through activities in the health care system. As an example, fetal malformation leading to death in most cases would not benefit from intervention, and pregnancy outcome could only be changed from perinatal death to termination if fetal diagnosis is available. Time of death can indicate cases that may have improved with health care, bearing in mind that intrapartum or neonatal death may also be averted through care activities in the antenatal period. Possible actions to avoid stillbirths in growth retarded fetuses are different from those related to normally grown stillborns.

This classification was used in a comparison between Sweden and Denmark (Langhoff-Roos et al., 1996), but has also been applied to perinatal deaths in the Baltic countries, the Moscow region, and Tashkent. An example from the comparison between

Lithuania and Scandinavia is given in table 2.5. The usefulness of the classification can be seen in that the relative increase in perinatal loss in Lithuania is different in the different groups. Attention is drawn to the doubled rate of perinatal loss from gross malformation, especially related to neural tube defects. It is also clear that an improvement in neonatal care would especially benefit babies with higher birthweights and longer gestations, which means that the improvements needed are not in the first place in high technology for the care of very premature babies, but are in the routine handling of more mature babies. It is interesting that in spite of intense efforts in Scandinavia to monitor what is considered to be high-risk pregnancies for intrauterine growth retardation, no differences are found in the risk of stillbirth with respect to the relative birthweight of the baby.

To further increase the understanding of factors involved in the prevention of perinatal death, a subgroup can be audited on a case-basis to define specific areas of substandard care or need for improvement. Such a comparison between Denmark and Sweden revealed a need for greater attention to the diagnosis of intrauterine asphyxia at admission to hospital in Denmark. A limitation of such case-based audits is that recommendations are based on possible or supposed benefit of a certain action in a limited number of cases with a bad outcome. Such a possible benefit will not necessarily mean that the screening or diagnostic procedure or the intervention is justified from a public health aspect, since the positive predictive value or the cost-effectiveness can be quite low on a population basis. Another objection to case-based perinatal audits is the risk that the reviewers are influenced by the knowledge of the bad outcome (Andersen, Hermann, and Gjorup, 1992). In that study, such a bias could not be demonstrated as related to knowledge of outcome.

One problem with assessment based on this type of grouping of perinatal deaths or case studies is that they do not take into account the background case-mix and complication rates in the population.

One way of overcoming this is to use the term "standard primi-para" and assess outcomes and use of health care procedures for the primipara without risk factors or complications at the start of labor (Swain et al., 1994). Increasingly, pregnancy outcome is also given as total fetal wastage, including late abortions and termina-tions based on fetal disease or malformation, since, from the point of view of the mother, these cases still have to be considered as pregnancy failures.

Many authors emphasize that an important aspect of quality of care is related to the patient–doctor relationship and the ability of the physician to involve the patient in the decision-making process (diMatteo, 1994). Also, these aspects of care can be audited and assessed, and are clearly related to outcome variables, such as patient satisfaction and level of information and acknowledge.

How can quality assurance change outcome?

For the process of quality assurance really to have an impact on the quality of care it is fundamental that it is not just an assessment of the quality indicators. The health staff has to be actively in-volved, and a feeling that this is a control system imposed from outside or above can be directly counterproductive to the objective of quality improvement (Ananijevic-Pandej, Cucic, and Doknic-Stefanovic, 1990; Morris, and Gambone, 1994).

How can a process of quality assurance contribute to improve pregnancy outcome? The first, very important factor is the setting of standards for quality of care in structure, process, and outcomes. If the standards are carefully adjusted to what is feasible and reasonable from the perspective of the health care providers, they will face a continuing challenge to meet the standards and a sense of achievement when the objectives are reached.

The clear definition of important outcomes and continuous registration of these outcomes has also proven to be efficient for quality improvement (Holthof, and Prins, 1993). These data will also provide a reliable source of information for decisionmakers on which to base changes in organization and structure and a tool for health advocates to use in public debate and political discussions. The quality assurance process will draw attention to the weak points in the health care system and question traditional health care procedures that are without scientific foundation (Munro, Reiter, and Gambone, 1994). Traditional practices without proven benefit, and which may even be harmful, are not uncommon in maternal and perinatal care. Many centers in Eastern Europe have been isolated from the active debate and the critical re-evaluation in this area that have taken place over the last few decades. Therefore, with increased awareness, resources can be reallocated and cost-effectiveness improved.

The ongoing dialogue with health care providers involves them in the quality assurance process and increases their motivation for their work and for the clients (Biswas et al., 1995; Harris, Yates, and Crosby, 1995). The various methods of involving clients or pregnant women and their experiences will often give a different perspective and result in a change in care in a favorable direction, often without extra costs and using fewer resources.

There are some obstacles in the introduction of a quality assurance process in settings where it is not integrated in the current system, which is the case in many Eastern European countries. Most individuals will react automatically with fear and suspicion to being assessed, and this is especially the case in an authoritarian system where a tradition of open discussion and criticism has not been common. Another problem is the lack of continuous, well-defined data recording, so the organization of such information collection systems is often the first step.

Conclusions

A process of quality assurance is the only way in which pregnancy outcome can be improved through health care activities. In addition, background factors of importance for adverse pregnancy outcome can be identified through quality assurance in health care and highlighted so that appropriate measures can be taken there as well as in other sectors of society. In this process, health workers at all levels are key participants and should actively take responsibility and be given ownership of the whole procedure.

References

Ananijevic-Pandej, J., Cucic, V., and Doknic-Stefanovic, D. 1990. Development of mechanisms for evaluation of the quality of perinatal care. *Yugoslav Gynecology and Perinatology* 30:39–41.

Andersen, K. V., Hermann, N., and Gjorup, T. 1992. Perinatal audit. Are experts biased by knowledge of outcome? A controlled study. *Danish Medical Bulletin* 39:197–9.

Biswas, A., Chew, S., Joseph, R., Arulkumaran, S., Anandakumar, C., and Ratnam, S. S. 1995. Towards improved perinatal care—perinatal audit. *Annals of the Academy of Medicine, Singapore* 24:211–7.

Buekens, P. 1990. Outcome measures of obstetrical and perinatal care. *Quality Assurance in Health Care* 2:253–262.

Cartlidge, P. H., Dawson, A. T., Stewart, J. H., and Vujanic, G. M. 1995. Value and quality of perinatal and infant postmortem examinations: cohort analysis of 400 consecutive deaths. *British Medical Journal*, 310:155–8.

Deming, W.E. 1986. *Out of crisis*. Cambridge, MA: MIT Center for Advanced Engineering Study.

diMatteo, M. R. 1994. The physician–patient relationship: effects of the quality of health care. *Clinical Obstetrics and Gynecology* 37:149–61.

Donabedian, A. 1978. The quality of medical care. *Science*, 200:854–6

Dunn, P. A., and McIlwaine, G. eds. *Perinatal audit—A report produced for the European Association of Perinatal Medicine*. 1996. New York and London: Parthenon.

Gaffney, G., Sellers, S., Flavell, V., Squier, M., and Johnson, A. 1994. Case-control study of intrapartum care, cerebral palsy, and perinatal death. *British Medical Journal* 308:743–50.

Hagerstrand, I., and Lundberg, L. M. 1993. The importance of post-mortem examinations of abortions and perinatal deaths. *Quality Assurance in Health Care* 5:295–7.

Hall, M. 1993. Audit of antenatal care. *Fetal and Maternal Medicine Review* 5:19–27.

Harris, J. K., Yates, B., and Crosby, W.M. 1995. A perinatal continuing education program: its effects on the knowledge and practices of health professionals. *Journal of Obstetric, Gynecological and Neonatal Nursing* 24:829–35.

Holthof, B., and Prins, P. 1993. Comparing hospital perinatal mortality rates: a quality improvement instrument. *Medical Care* 31:801–7.

Hutchon, D. J. 1996. A method of proportional audit of perinatal care. *British Journal of Obstetrics and Gynaecology* 103:402–4.

Jahn, A., and Berle, P. 1996. Quality of prenatal data in the Hessian Perinatal Registry. A comparison with data from maternal health record and results of a pregnancy survey. *Geburtshilfe und Frauenheilkunde* 56:132–8.

Jahrig, K., Jahrig, D., and Heinrich, J. 1988. Quality assessment in neonatology. *Zentralblatt für Gynäkologie* 110:1473–84.

Langhoff-Roos, J., Borch-Christensen, H., Larsen, S., Lindberg, B., and Wennergren, M. 1996. Potentially avoidable perinatal deaths in Denmark and Sweden 1991. *Acta Obstetricia et Gynecologica Scandinavica* 75: 820–5.

Loegering, L., Reiter, R. C., and Gambone, J. C. 1994. Measuring the quality of health care. *Clinical Obstetrics and Gynecology* 37:122–36.

Maresh, M., and Hall, M. 1991. *Second bulletin*, Manchester, UK: Royal College of Obstetricians and Gynaecologists Medical Audit Unit.

Meeker, C. I. 1994. Quality improvement: then and now. *Clinical Obstetrics and Gynecology* 37:115–21.

Morris, M., and Gambone, J.C. 1994. Making continual improvements to health care. *Clinical Obstetrics and Gynecology* 37:137–48.

Munro, M. G., Reiter, R. C., and Gambone, J. C. 1994. Technology assessment in women's health care. *Clinical Obstetrics and Gynecology* 37:180–91.

Shaw, C. D. 1990. Perioperative and perinatal death as measures for quality assurance. *Quality Assurance in Health Care* 2:235–41.

Sokol, R. J., Chik, L., and Zador, I. 1992. Approaching the millennium: perinatal problems and software solutions. *Early Human Development* 29:51–6.

33

Swain, S., Agrawal, A., Bhatia, B. D., and Rajaram, P. 1994. Audit in maternal and child health. *Indian Pediatrics* 31:1397–402

WHO. 1995. *The OBSQUID Project. Quality Development in Perinatal Care.* Final report. Copenhagen: World Health Organization.

WHO Regional Office for Europe and United Nations Population Fund. 1995. *Family planning and reproductive health in CCEE/NIS.* DOC. EUR/ICP/ FMLY 94 03/PB01. Copenhagen: World Health Organization.

Wiegers, T. A., Keirse, M. J., Berghs, G. A., and vad der Zee, J. 1996. An approach to measuring quality of midwifery care. *Journal of Clinical Epidemiology* 49:319–25.

Table 2.1

American College of Obstetricians and Gynecologists Obstetric Clinical Indicators

Maternal indicators

Maternal mortality

Unplanned readmission within 14 days

Cardiopulmonary arrest

In-hospital initiation of antibiotics 24 hours or more after term vaginal delivery

Unplanned removal, injury, or repair of organ during operative procedure

In-hospital maternal red blood cell transfusion or hematocrit < 22 vol% or hemoglobin of < 7.0 g or decrease in hematocrit of 11 vol% or hemoglobin of 3.5 g or more

Maternal length of stay more than 5 days after vaginal delivery or more than 7 days after cesarean delivery

Eclampsia

Delivery unattended by the "responsible" physician[a]

Postpartum return to delivery room or operating room for management

Induction of labor for an indication other than diabetes, premature rupture of membranes, pregnancy-induced hypertension, postterm gestation, intrauterine growth retardation, cardiac disease, isoimmunization, fetal demise, or chorioamnionitis

Cesarean delivery required

Primary cesarean delivery for fetal distress

Primary cesarean delivery for failure to progress

Delivery of an infant with a birthweight < 2500 g or respiratory distress syndrome following induction of labor

Neonatal indicators

Perinatal mortality of a fetus or infant surviving less than 28 days and weighing 500 g or more at delivery

Intrapartum death, in hospital, or a fetus or infant weighing 500 g or more

Neonatal mortality of an inborn infant with a birthweight of 750–999 g in an institution with a neonatal intensive care unit[b]

Delivery of an infant weighing < 1800 g in an institution without a neonatal intensive care unit

Transfer of a neonate to a neonatal intensive care unit in another institution

Term infant admitted to a neonatal intensive care unit

Apgar score of 4 or less at 5 minutes

Birth trauma (#767 in ICD-9 directory), such as shoulder dystocia, cephalohematoma, Erb's palsy, and clavicular fracture but not caput

Diagnosis of fetal "massive aspiration syndrome (#770.1 in ICD-9-CM)"

Inborn term infant with clinically apparent seizures recorded before discharge

---

[a] To be defined by each institution.

[b] An inborn infant is one born in this hospital rather than one transferred from another institution.

Table 2.2

Key common European quality development indicators
in perinatal care (OBSQUID project)

1. Intrauterine deaths (22–27 completed weeks)
2. Antenatal deaths (after 27 completed weeks)
3. Fetal deaths in partum
4. Deaths within 0–6 days after birth
5. Deaths within 7–27 days after birth
6. Born before/at 31 completed weeks
7. Born between 32 and 36 completed weeks
8. Major congenital malformations
9. Apgar score ≤ 6 at 5 minutes
10. Infants with respiratory distress syndrome
11. Neonatal seizures within 7 days
12. Maternal deaths
13. Hysterectomy within 2 days after delivery
14. Women with blood transfusion
15. Eclampsia in pregnancy
16. Women with multiple pregnancies
17. Multiple pregnancies detected before delivery
18. Parturients with no prenatal visits before birth
19. Unattended births
20. Cesarian sections
21. Forceps/vacuum extractions

Table 2.3

Perinatal mortality in the year 1995 in Tallinn, Tartu, and Estonia, using different birthweight cutoff points (Courtesy Dr. H. Karro)

	Tallinn Pelgulinna Maternity Hospital	Tallinn Central Hospital	Tartu Women's Clinic	Estonia
Stillborns ≥ 500 g	21 11.3‰	19 8.2‰	16 8.6‰	99 7.3‰
Stillborns ≥ 1000 g	11 5.9‰	14 6.0‰	8 4.3‰	70 5.2‰
0-6 days ≥ 500 g	19 10.2‰	41 17.6‰	11 5.9‰	103 7.6‰
0-6 days ≥ 1000 g	13 7.0‰	24 10.3‰	7 3.8‰	69 5.1‰
Perinatal mortality rate ≥ 500 g	40 21.6‰	60 25.8‰	27 14.6‰	202 15.0‰
Perinatal mortality rate ≥ 1000 g	24 12.9‰	38 16.3‰	15 8.1‰	139 10.3‰

Table 2.4

Common Nordic–Baltic perinatal death classification

   I. Fetal malformation
  II. Antenatal death; single growth-retarded fetus, ≥ 28 weeks of gestation
 III. Antenatal death; single fetus, ≥ 28 weeks of gestation
(IV. Antenatal death; before 28 weeks of gestation.)
  V. Antenatal death; multiple pregnancy
 VI. Intrapartum death after admission (≥ 28 weeks of gestation)
(VII. Intrapartum death after admission [before 28 weeks of gestation.])
VIII. Neonatal death; 28–33 weeks of gestation and Apgar score > 6 after 5 minutes
 IX. Neonatal death; 28–33 weeks of gestation and Apgar score > 7 after 5 minutes
  X. Neonatal death; ≥ 34 weeks of gestation and Apgar score > 6 after 5 minutes
 XI. Neonatal death; ≥ 34 weeks of gestation and Apgar score < 7 after 5 minutes
XII. Neonatal death; before 28 weeks of gestation
XIII. Unclassified

Table 2.5

Perinatal deaths by categories of the Nordic–Baltic perinatal death classification
in Lithuania 1993–94 (N=1127) and Denmark and Sweden 1991 (N=1282)

Category	Lithuania 1993–94		Denmark and Sweden 1991		Odds ratio and 99% confidence interval	
	N	Rate (/10 000)	N	Rate (/10 000)		
I	296	32.8	305	16.2	2.03	(1.64 to 2.49)
II	90	10.0	150	8.0	1.25	(0.88 to 2.49)
III	162	18.0	398	21.1	0.85	(0.66 to 1.08)
V	11	1.2	55	2.9	0.42	(0.17 to 0.97)
VI	88	9.8	50	2.7	3.67	(2.32 to 5.79)
VIII	88	9.8	42	2.2	4.37	(2.69 to 7.08)
IX	89	9.9	39	2.1	4.76	(2.90 to 7.81)
X	49	5.4	22	1.2	4.65	(2.39 to 9.00)
XI	54	6.0	41	2.2	2.75	(1.61 to 4.68)
XII	144	16.0	175	9.3	1.72	(1.28 to 2.29)
XIII	56	6.2	5	0.3		

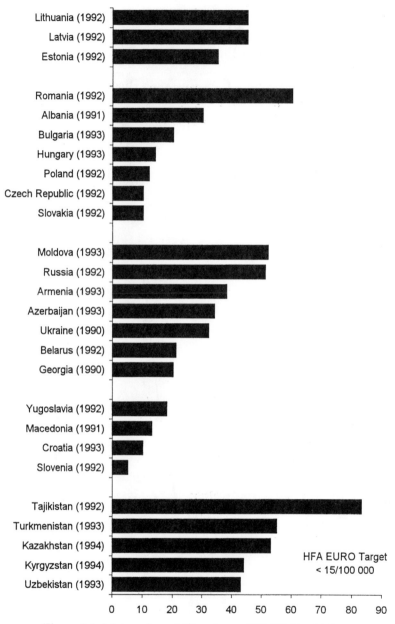

Figure 2.1. Maternal mortality rate per 100 000 live births.
Source: WHO/EURO/SFPU/avril 1995.

39

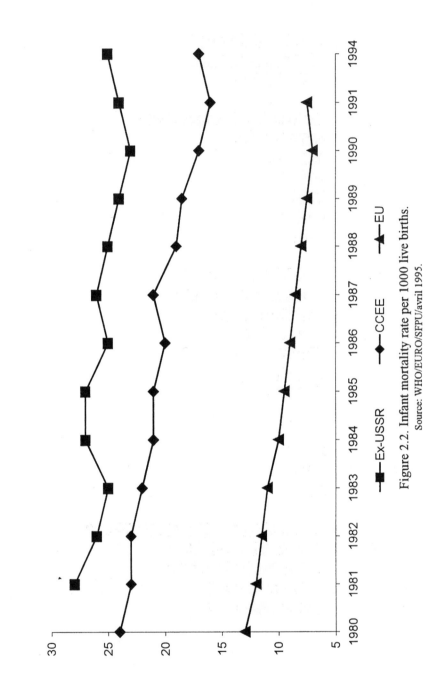

Figure 2.2. Infant mortality rate per 1000 live births.
Source: WHO/EURO/SFPU/avril 1995.

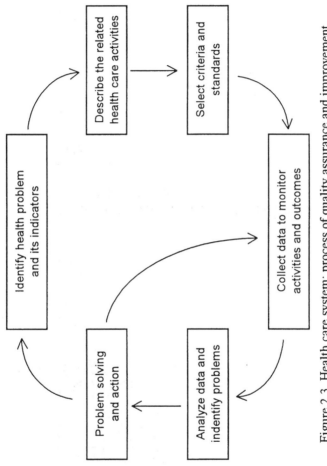

Figure 2.3. Health care system: process of quality assurance and improvement.

41

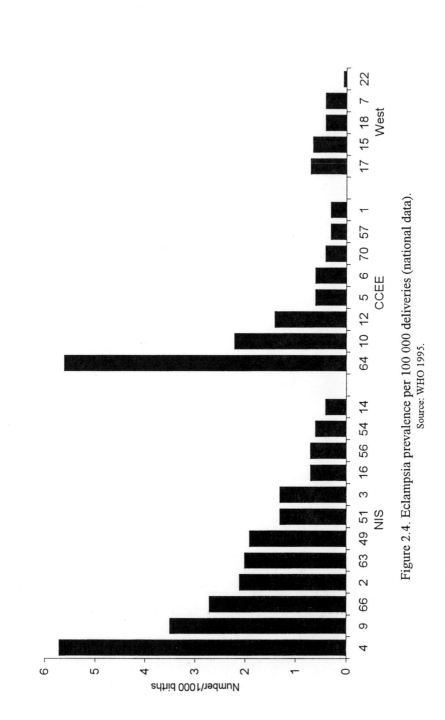

Figure 2.4. Eclampsia prevalence per 100 000 deliveries (national data).
Source: WHO 1995.

42

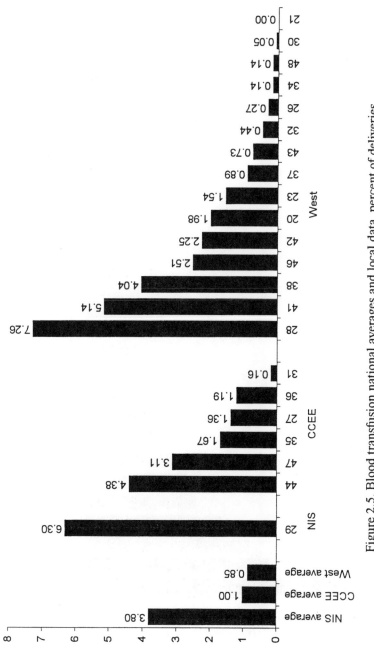

Figure 2.5. Blood transfusion national averages and local data, percent of deliveries.
Source: WHO 1995.

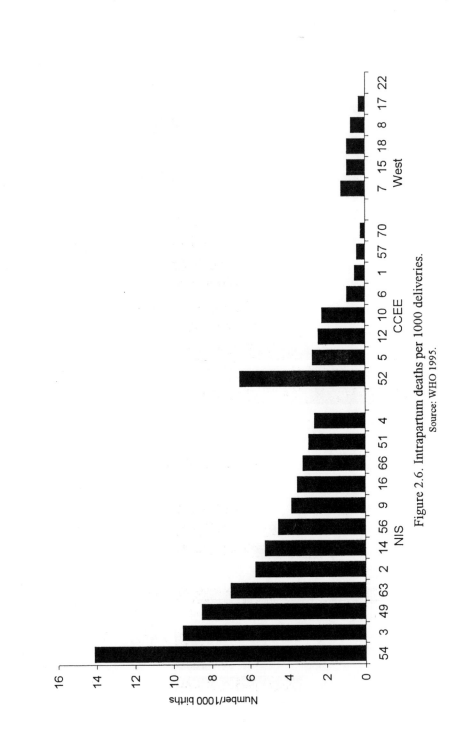

Figure 2.6. Intrapartum deaths per 1000 deliveries.
Source: WHO 1995.

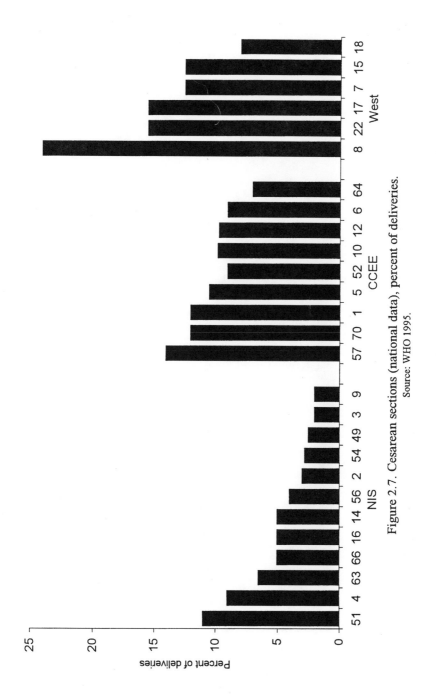

Figure 2.7. Cesarean sections (national data), percent of deliveries.
Source: WHO 1995.

The challenge of rising trends in the incidence of sexually transmitted diseases in Eastern Europe*

A. GROMYKO

WHO Regional Office for Europe, Copenhagen, Denmark

Abstract

An alarming rise in sexually transmitted diseases (STDs) has been observed in the Newly Independent States of Eastern Europe during the last few years. While during 1989–92 the incidence of syphilis in countries in Western Europe decreased to a level below 2 per 100 000 population, there has been an extremely rapid rise in the official notifications of syphilis in the Russian Federation, Ukraine, Moldova, Belarus, and some other Newly Independent States, up to the level 100–170 per 100 000 population. This represents a thirty- to fortyfold increase from 1989 to 1995. The break up of the USSR and the transition to market reforms have caused enormous political, economic, and social changes, which has had a tremendous influence on the sexual behavior of the population.

On the other side, the obsolete treatment regimens, unfavorable legislation, little primary prevention, and, consequently, the low

* The article is based on the data reported to WHO by the National Health Authorities, on the report of the WHO Mission to Russia on assessment of the STD situation in December 1995 (WHO/EURO, unpublished document) and on the report of the WHO Meeting "Epidemic of sexually transmitted diseases in Eastern Europe" held in WHO/EURO in May 1996 (WHO/EURO, 1996, Document EUR/ICP/CMDS 08 01 01).

level of health seeking behavior have favored the increasing length of time when infected patients remain untreated and thus continue to spread infections. In response to the epidemic, WHO convened a meeting of experts from the countries most affected. The participants called for urgent action, including a careful assessment of existing systems for controlling the spread of STDs, reallocation of resources among the various activity areas, and strongly advocated generating awareness at the top level of government to strengthen its support for the recommended initiatives. They also urged better national coordination of programs to promote sexual health and prevent STDs and human immunodeficiency virus infection, that statutory services be made more acceptable and affordable for patients, and that efforts be made to ensure that all health workers managing patients with STDs, including those in the private sector, provide high quality care.

Introduction

At the same time as Western Europe has witnessed a significant decline in the incidence of syphilis and gonorrhea, there has been an extremely rapid rise—of syphilis especially—in the eastern part of Europe. During the years 1980–93 the incidence of syphilis in the countries of Western Europe dropped to below 2 per 100 000 persons and the incidence of gonorrhea to 20 per 100 000. But since 1989 there has been an extremely rapid rise, particularly in the Newly Independent States (NIS), in the notification rate of syphilis. In the Russian Federation, for example, the incidence was 86 per 100 000 in 1994 and 172.1 in 1995, which represents a fortyfold increase from 1989 to 1995. In general terms, in many countries of the former USSR the incidence of syphilis has increased 15–30 times, from 5–15 per 100 000 as observed in 1990 to as high as 120–170 per 100 000 in 1995. An incidence rate higher than 50 per 100 000 population was reported in 1995 in all the Baltic states (fig. 3.1), in Belarus, Kazakhstan, Kyrgyzstan, the Republic of Moldova, and Ukraine (figs. 3.2, 3.3, 3.4).

In urban areas and in some provinces of the northwestern part of the Russian Federation the incidence rate of syphilis in 1995 was at the level of 300–400 per 100 000 population. Figures 3.5, 3.6, 3.7 show the absolute numbers of notified cases of syphilis in several NIS, illustrating the dramatic level of the epidemic. Neighboring countries have recorded the importation of sexually transmitted diseases (STDs) from the countries of the former USSR. Finland, particularly, has experienced an increased importation of gonorrhea from Russia and Estonia (fig. 3.8). An outbreak of syphilis related to the importation of the disease from Russia has recently also been identified in Finland, and consequently the downward trend in the incidence of cases of syphilis observed in Finland during the last 10 years has started to revert upwards in 1995 (fig. 3.9).

Origins of the syphilis epidemic

The occurrence of curable bacterial STDs in the population is determined by the biological characteristics of the organisms, the efficacy of medical interventions on the transmissibility and natural history of the infection, and by patterns of sexual behavior. The number of partners in unprotected sexual intercourse has an impact on the risk of transmission. Medical management of cases and their sexual partners reduces the length of time in which the individual remains infected.

The current process of rapid change in the Russian Federation has, among other things, caused a decline in the gross domestic product by an average of 12% per year in real terms during 1990–94, with a massive increase in differences in income, poverty, unemployment, and migration. These recent developments have a substantial impact on the structure, availability, and effectiveness of health services as well as on sexual behavior.

Tremendous social and economic upheaval throughout Eastern Europe during the last 10 years has followed in the wake of the transition to a market economy. The wide-ranging political, economic, and social changes that have taken place in countries of the former USSR over the last 5 years as they emerge from the fragmentation of the country have provided the soil within which the observed epidemics have grown. The major economic downturns have very damaging social consequences; in many of these countries there is, for instance, general instability in society and breakdown of social infrastructures; war and civilian and ethnic conflicts; sharp increases in migration; and large numbers of refugees and homeless and unemployed persons.

All of these factors have very negative effects on the incidence of "social" diseases, such as tuberculosis, STDs, scabies, and psychiatric illnesses among many others. Simple economic factors are also very important: more than 30 million people in the Russian Federation now live below the poverty level. The physical and moral condition of youth, especially, has weakened significantly due to malnourishment, the increase in alcohol consumption and smoking, and early sexual promiscuity, accompanied by violence and increasing child prostitution. As might be expected, these social developments have had considerable repercussions on the health of the population, particularly on trends for curable STDs.

Curable STDs are not only a concern because of the discomfort caused by the acute infection. They can have very damaging consequences, including infertility, ectopic pregnancy, urethral stricture, cervical cancer, premature mortality, congenital syphilis, fetal wastage, low birthweight, premature delivery, ophthalmia neonatorum, and other complications. What is more, they are proven risk factors in the transmission of the human immunodeficiency virus (HIV), and therefore control is a major concern in preventing the spread of HIV and AIDS.

It is clear that practically all of the NIS are experiencing a major epidemic of STDs, especially syphilis, and that younger people and adolescents are affected to a greater extent than older age groups. The origins of these epidemics can be traced not only to the social causes already mentioned, but also to the accessibility, acceptability, and effectiveness of control mechanisms. These factors hold the key to bringing the epidemics under control.

The areas of strength and weakness of existing systems must be recognized and steps taken to improve the balance between different areas of activity. Strong representations must be made to the highest levels of government to generate awareness of the problem and to secure support for the recommended initiatives.

The WHO Regional Office for Europe organized an action-oriented meeting of experts from the countries concerned with three expert advisers. They sought to exchange up-to-date information from each country on the extent of the problem, identify priority actions to control the epidemic, specify technical support and training needs, and agree on an overall plan of action.

Directions for the control of the epidemic

Prevention and promotion of sexual health

The absence of effective national coordination of programs of health promotion in the area of sexual health and STD prevention is perhaps the most serious shortcoming in the existing situation. Governments urgently need to bring together all agencies concerned to develop a strategy rapidly to implement the promotion of sexual health. Such a strategy would:

• integrate existing health promotion activities within dermatology–venereology and HIV/AIDS programs;

• be targeted at youth from a young age, at groups at high risk of infection, including homosexual men, prostitutes and their clients, and other socially vulnerable groups;

• use effective techniques of mass information, peer education, and face-to-face counseling, and involve key opinion leaders within communities.

Clinical services

Clinical services are faced with both increasing workloads and shrinking resources. Moreover, traditional health care practices, relying frequently on inpatient management and requiring patients to identify themselves and to accept strict legal obligations are proving unworkable. Patients are increasingly unwilling to accept such conditions and as a result there is a rapid growth in the provision of care outside the law by both medical and nonmedical practitioners, as well as of self-treatment. It is thus a priority to make state services more accessible and acceptable to patients. This can be done by:

• allowing patients to choose where they will be treated;

• introducing without delay a fully anonymous system of care, where patients are not required to identify themselves for either diagnosis or treatment;

• changing from inpatient to outpatient care, especially for treatment of syphilis;

• improving case management in general; for instance, with same-day treatment, simplification of follow-up, the use of diagnostic tests within the context of simplified case management algorithms based on clinical features of the disease, use of generic drugs where possible, and developing ways to ensure that contacts and sexual partners seek examination and treatment;

• providing affordable or free services.

The general consensus was that clinical services are well provided with expertise but often sorely lack funding, which requires action by governments and other responsible authorities.

Management of STDs
by non-dermatologists–venereologists

Since this is the current situation, efforts should be made to try to ensure that all persons handling patients with STDs provide quality care; for instance, by introducing licensing systems.

Training

While training of dermatologists–venereologists is of a high standard, in order to make clinical management more effective training in dermatology–venereology could be modified to place more emphasis on health promotion, positive doctor–patient relationships, and patients' rights. Also, keeping point (3) in mind, dermatologists–venereologists and their organizations need to find ways to share their knowledge and expertise more effectively with other clinical colleagues who are likely to see patients with STDs.

Active case finding and screening

Since active efforts to identify individuals with STDs provide comparatively reliable data on the incidence of syphilis, the screening of pregnant women and other clinical and occupational groups under existing programs should be maintained or extended, while fully respecting the rights of patients.

Surveillance

Changing epidemiological circumstances and patterns of health care require a review of existing services. *(a)* Notification of cases should be anonymous. *(b)* Pilot sentinel surveillance schemes should be introduced and evaluated in individual dermatology–venereology clinics, in an attempt to obtain more epidemiological information. *(c)* More general implementation of sentinel surveillance should be considered.

Developing better lines of communication between health professionals in various disciplines, governmental and nongovernmental organizations, the general population, and high-risk groups is an urgent priority and will likely require innovative action. Existing laws concerning the control of sexually transmitted diseases are by and large of little use in controlling epidemics such as the ones now developing in Eastern Europe. Changes are urgently needed, both to make the law less oppressive and at the same time to protect the rights of individuals who may be at risk of infection from others known to have STDs. Finally, ways need to be found to allow countries to share their experiences of developing and implementing programs and innovations, perhaps by creating a regional organization for STD control in Eastern Europe under the auspices of international health organizations.

Conclusions

Most of the NIS of Eastern Europe are experiencing major epidemics of sexually transmitted diseases, especially of syphilis, mostly affecting young people and adolescents. The epidemics appear to be rooted in the rapid economic and social changes that have occurred in recent years and the effect of the changes on sexual behavior and attitudes and the acceptability and effectiveness of clinical services. Action needs to be taken to control these epidemics, such as careful assessment of the weaknesses and strengths within the existing systems for STD control and reallocation of resources among the various activity areas. Strong advocacy addressing the top level of government is required to generate awareness of the problem and to strengthen political commitment and support for the recommended initiatives.

The absence of effective national coordination of programs of health promotion in the area of sexual health and STD/HIV prevention is the most important shortcoming of the existing situation. Clinical services are faced with increasing workloads and shrinking resources. The traditional form of case management, characterized by frequent inpatient care regimens, registration of personal data with a lack of confidentiality and anonymity, and strong legal obligations imposed on the patient, is becoming impractical and inefficient. Patients are increasingly unwilling to accept such conditions and there is consequently a rapid growth in provision of care by medical and nonmedical practitioners outside the regulated statutory services and of self-treatment.

Consequently, a priority is to make statutory services more accessible and acceptable to patients. Since management of STDs by non-dermatologists–venereologists is a reality, it is necessary to ensure that all those managing patients with STDs provide a high standard of care. Training of dermatologists–venereologists and other professionals concerned with sexual health is in general of high standard, but the recommendations listed above will generate a need for additional training to introduce more rational approaches in clinical management and health promotion within STD clinics.

Active case finding and screening are efficient approaches for identifying substantial numbers of individuals with STDs, especially those with syphilis. Existing surveillance systems have served well, but changing epidemiological circumstances and changing patterns of health care require review of the systems and new initiatives. The present legislation related to STD control was considered largely unhelpful in controlling the current epidemics.

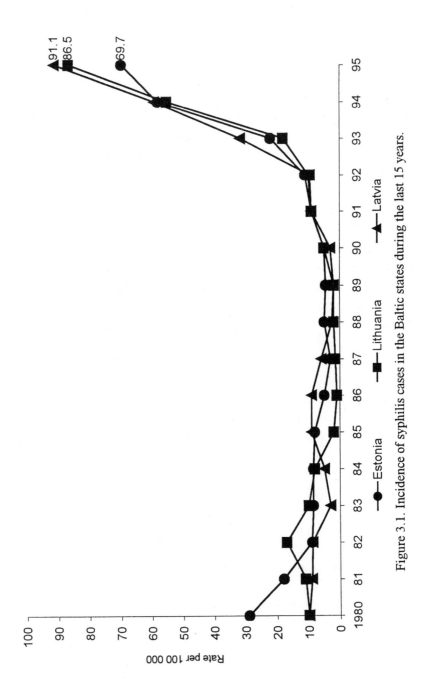

Figure 3.1. Incidence of syphilis cases in the Baltic states during the last 15 years.

56

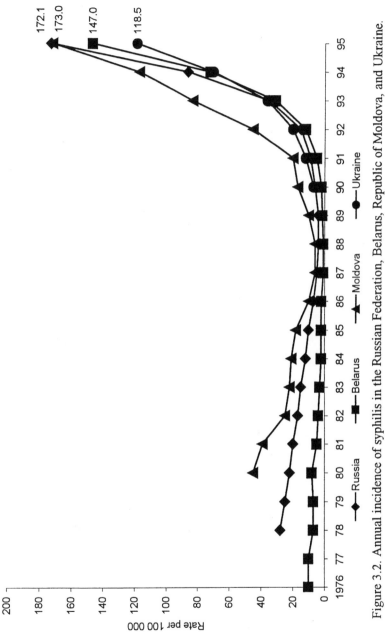

Figure 3.2. Annual incidence of syphilis in the Russian Federation, Belarus, Republic of Moldova, and Ukraine.

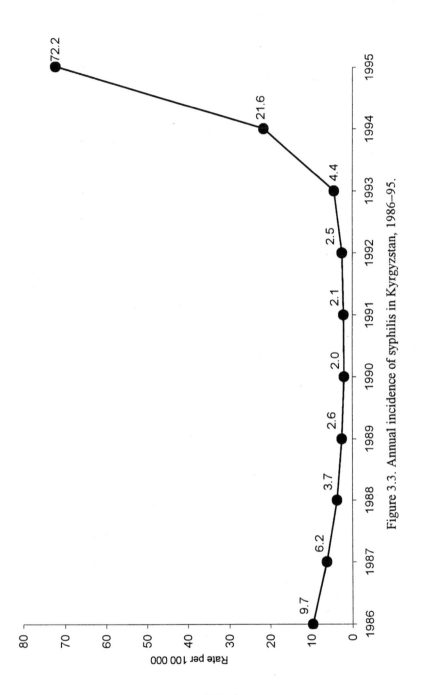

Figure 3.3. Annual incidence of syphilis in Kyrgyzstan, 1986–95.

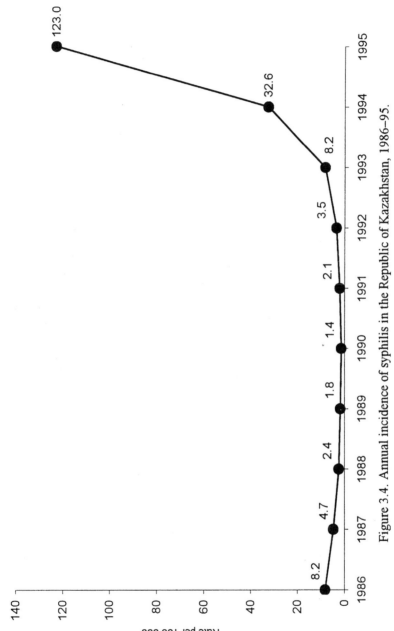

Figure 3.4. Annual incidence of syphilis in the Republic of Kazakhstan, 1986–95.

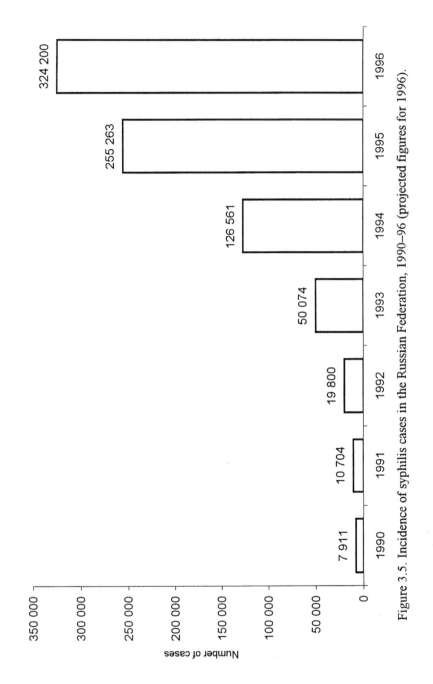

Figure 3.5. Incidence of syphilis cases in the Russian Federation, 1990–96 (projected figures for 1996).

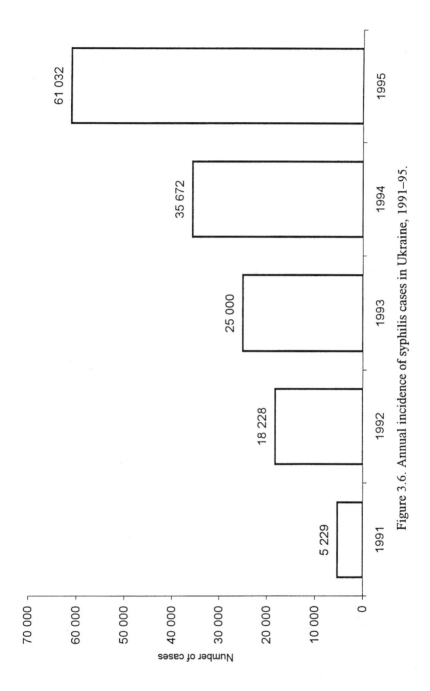

Figure 3.6. Annual incidence of syphilis cases in Ukraine, 1991–95.

61

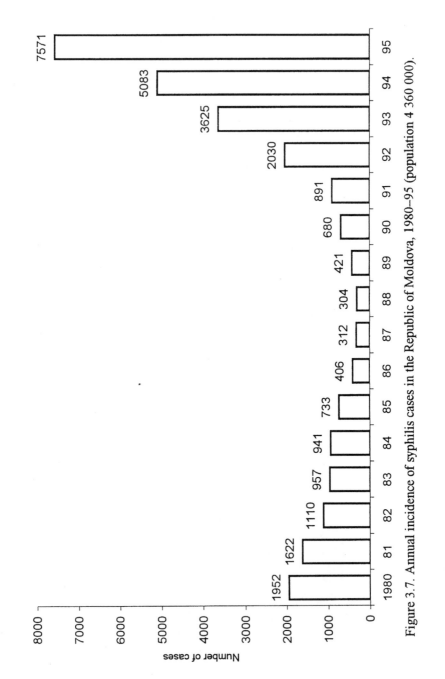

Figure 3.7. Annual incidence of syphilis cases in the Republic of Moldova, 1980–95 (population 4 360 000).

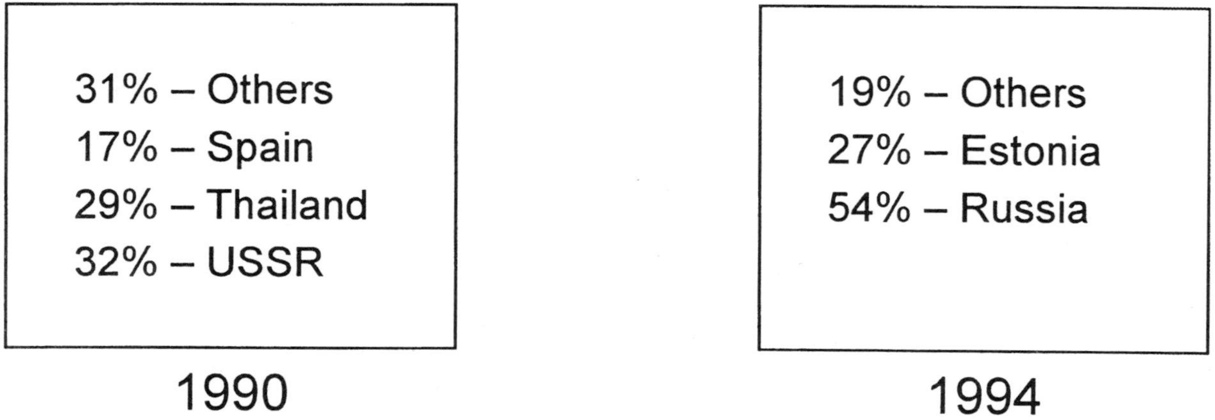

1994

19% – Others
27% – Estonia
54% – Russia

1990

31% – Others
17% – Spain
29% – Thailand
32% – USSR

Figure 3.8. Imported cases of gonorrhea in Helsinki. Helsinki City STD Clinic (42% of cases reported in 1994 were imported).

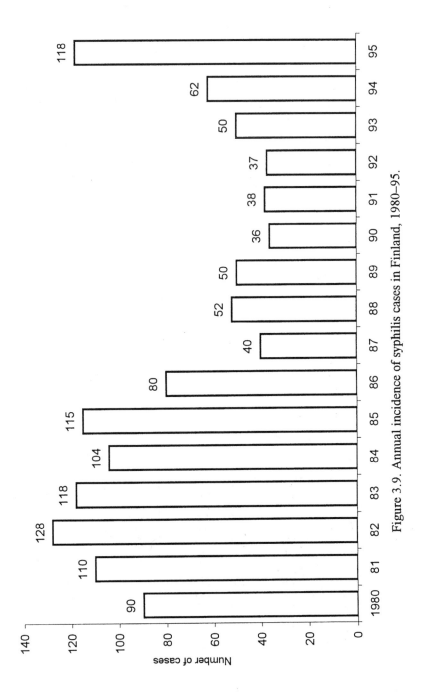

Figure 3.9. Annual incidence of syphilis cases in Finland, 1980–95.

Obstacles and opportunities in the development of adolescent reproductive health care

GUNTA LAZDANE and ILONA AUZINA

Department of Obstetrics and Gynecology, Medical Academy of Latvia, Riga, Latvia

Abstract

Family planning and reproductive health in the countries of Central and Eastern Europe and the Newly Independent States of the former USSR are in a stage of transition, as almost every area of life has been in these countries since they regained independence. While conditions for women's health are generally improving, there are a lot of problems concerning adolescents (aged 10–19 years). The psychological status of young people is influenced by the atmosphere in the family and society and by the economic downturn.

A large proportion of all induced abortions in the countries of Eastern Europe is in the age group 19 years and younger. Adolescents delivered 19% of all babies in Latvia in 1995. There is a tremendous increase in the incidence of sexually transmitted diseases in most of the countries of Eastern Europe, which has a great influence on the reproductive health of the population, especially teenagers. The number of sex workers has grown over the last few years and 10% of prostitutes in Latvia are adolescents.

Sex education is taught in every fourth school in Latvia. However, there is no unified training for teachers, nor is there an accepted teaching program for all years. There is only one youth health center in Latvia (with a population of 2.6 million) where young people can attend health services for their reproductive health and sex life. A special lecture course is delivered to young people there, aimed at helping adolescents to understand themselves better.

To a great extent, information and education in Eastern European countries are provided by nongovernmental organizations and their volunteers. There should be governmental support for preventive activities in reproductive health for adolescents.

Introduction

In Eastern European countries the reproductive health needs of adolescents are largely ignored by the current reproductive health services, although the importance of adolescence as a stage of development in the life of the individual has recently received international recognition. The Program of Action of the International Conference on Population and Development held in 1994 in Cairo stated: "Governments, in collaboration with non-governmental organisations, are urged to establish programmes to meet the needs of adolescents and address adolescent sexual and reproductive health issues, including unwanted pregnancy, unsafe abortion, sexually transmitted diseases and HIV/AIDS" (UN, 1995).

Adolescents comprise a large proportion of the world's population. In many countries they make up 20–25% of the population (Fathalla et al., 1990). Many nongovernmental organizations have selected young people as the target group of their activities. As a nongovernmental federation of voluntary associations, the International Planned Parenthood Federation declares in its Strategic Plan—Vision 2000: "... institutional barriers continue to obstruct the provision of effective programmes that could not only prevent the rising incidence of adolescent pregnancy, abortion and sexually transmitted diseases, but could also help young people to realise their sexuality in a positive and responsible manner."

Eastern European countries have embarked on a difficult process of transition from an authoritarian political system to democracy, from centrally guided economies to open market systems, from abortion to contraception, and from ignorance to knowledge. This transition period has created changes in the political life and economy of the country, in the lifestyle, priorities, and living standards of the people. Many people have encountered difficulties in coping with the transition, but young people are a particularly vulnerable group.

Since the restoration of full independence in 1991, Latvia belongs to the group of countries with economies in transition. Latvia can be used as a typical example of the processes influencing the lifestyle and the reproductive health of adolescents.

Political and economic situation in Latvia

In Latvia in 1994, 13.5% of the estimated population of 2.6 million (1993) were adolescents. In 1995, the income per capita in Latvia was 37 Lats ($=0.55 Ls) and Latvian trade unions estimated that in 1995 the cost of food in Latvia was 31 Ls (UNDP, 1996). A survey of household budgets indicated that the poorest spent only one-fifth of the amount spent by the rich on food (UNDP, 1995). Large families encountered the greatest difficulties.

Thus, it is not surprising that the birthrate has decreased and that in 1995 population growth was negative: −7.4 per 1000 inhabitants. These difficult times have also led to a lower birthrate in most Eastern European countries. In April 1996, 7.0% of the economically active population in Latvia were registered as unemployed. Officials believe that "hidden unemployment," caused by work stoppages, unpaid leave, and a reduction in the work week, may affect an additional 6–7% of the population.

With the economic recession, the number of families (single parents, families with many children, the unemployed, alcoholics, drug addicts, and families with a disabled or seriously ill child) that are unable or unwilling to take care of their children has grown. On 1 July 1995 about one-sixth of the population of Riga (132 754) people were registered as indigent by social assistance agencies (*Health in Riga,* 1996). From infancy to adolescence children in such families encounter serious problems such as poverty, alcoholism, and violence. In addition, 10% of convicted persons are under the age of 18 (fig. 4.1.) and they obtain their "sex education" in prison or in special institutions. In 1995 there were 6511 children with no parental support or supervision. These factors influence the level of education. Also in 1995, 2500 children of school age did not attend school in Latvia (fig. 4.2). In the school year 1994–95, 6% of children in class 9 were expelled from school.

The social environment affects the process of psychological changes in adolescents. One in four children in Latvia is born outside marriage (fig. 4.3) and nearly two-thirds of all marriages in Latvia end in divorce. The proportion of children born to unmarried mothers has increased in all Eastern European countries. This was greatest in Estonia, where 41% of all new mothers in 1994 were unmarried compared to only 25% in 1989. In Hungary the proportion increased from 12.4% in 1989 to 19.3% in 1994, in Poland from 5.8 to 9%, and in Russia from 13.5 to 19% (Karlen, and Hagner, 1996). All these social and economic problems directly influence the reproductive health of adolescents . Unfortunately, not all of these problems are studied or registered by the authorities and no data are available. This paper will focus on the trends in adolescent pregnancy and the incidence of sexually transmitted diseases in Latvia today.

Teenage pregnancy

There are no data on the average of the first sexual experience of adolescents in Latvia. However, the average age at first sexual intercourse among 200 women attending the contraceptive clinic in Latvia and participating in a collaborative study with the Institute of Clinical Bacteriology, Uppsala University, was 18.97 (standard deviation 0.14 years) (in Sweden: mean 16.01, SD 0.13 years).

There is a trend toward an increase in teenage pregnancies in Latvia. Most of these pregnancies are unwanted and unplanned. In the age group 19 years and younger, 20–30% of first pregnancies result in induced abortion. In 1995, 14.5% of all induced abortions (25 933) in Latvia were among teenagers (fig. 4.4), and this percentage is increasing from year to year. Of these abortions, 24% (64 cases) were carried out after the twelfth week of gestation, and there were two cases of criminal, unsafe abortions in this age group in 1995 as well as in 1996. If we summarize all types of abortions (including spontaneous) among teenagers, almost 3000 pregnancies in this age group end in abortion every year in Latvia (2952 cases in 1994, 3146 in 1995, 3159 in 1996).

The total number of deliveries in Latvia in 1995 was 21 620 and the birthrate has been decreasing since 1991. There were 3262 deliveries by mothers 19 years and younger (10 were under 14 years of age) in 1994 and 3114 (12) in 1995, (fig. 4.5.). There are a few small studies of the course of pregnancy and delivery in this age group in Latvia. In one study, of 306 adolescent mothers who delivered at the Riga Maternity Hospital in 1995 (Miltina et al., 1996), 55% were unmarried, 69% had no occupation, 31% attended an antenatal clinic for the first time after 22 weeks of gestation, 14% were multigravidae, and 10% multiparae. There was a higher incidence of urogenital tract infections and anemia in comparison with 300 cases aged of 20–25 years. There were 7.5% premature deliveries (5.1% in the control group) in the teenage group.

There are registered maternal deaths in mothers 19 years and younger in Latvia: one death in 1991, two in 1994, and one in 1995. Negative social, physical, and psychological factors are all associated with adolescent pregnancy. As teenage pregnancies occur more frequently among young women from lower social strata, it has often been explained that the poorer outcomes of those pregnancies were due to social characteristics rather than to the young age of the mother. However, recent studies aimed at disentangling the different factors behind the adverse outcome of teenage pregnancies have indicated an independent negative impact of young maternal age (Chenet, 1996).

Sexually transmitted diseases among adolescents

Sexual activity among adolescents is increasing worldwide. Early sexual intercourse results in an increased risk of sexually transmitted diseases (STDs). Sexual intercourse at a very young age has also been associated with an increased risk of cervical cancer. In the past few years there has been a dramatic increase in the total number of cases of STDs in Latvia, and the average age of the patients suffering from STDs is decreasing. Morbidity from syphilis increased by 30% over the first 9 months in 1996 in comparison with 1995, and up to 10% of these patients are adolescents (fig. 4.6). The same trends are apparent in the incidence rates for gonorrhea and chlamydia infection (fig. 4.7).

Sexual violence to young women

In many societies, adolescents face pressures to engage in sexual activity. Young women, particularly adolescents from low-income homes, are especially vulnerable. According to the data of the Moral Police of Latvia, one in ten registered prostitutes in Latvia is a teenager (fig. 4.8) and they are typically poorly informed about how to protect themselves. In 1995 the youngest case of sexually transmitted syphilis in Latvia was a 12-year-old girl. Similar to the situation in the whole of the former communist bloc, sexual molestation of children has been a virtually forbidden topic of discussion. Consequently, the lack of experience and knowledge among the police and social services is a great obstacle to dealing with this. For the same reason, no facts or statistics have been compiled. There are no data on sexual violence in the family, but when the number of articles in newspapers and journals dedicated to this topic are analyzed it indicates that the number of cases are increasing.

Adolescent contraception

The number of people using modern, effective methods of contraception is low in the countries of Eastern Europe. In accordance with the data of the Bureau of Medical Statistics of the Latvia Republic (Republic of Latvia, 1996), only 19% of women of childbearing age (15–44 years) used combined oral contraception, an intrauterine device, or had surgical sterilization performed. The contraceptive prevalence rate is estimated at 23% in Estonia (1994), 11% in Romania (1992), and 59% in the Czech Republic (1994) (WHO and UN Population Fund, 1995). There are no data on condom use in Latvia or on contraceptive use among adolescents. In 1994 and 1995, 3121 adolescents consulted a gynecologist for family planning counseling (Zumente, 1996). In 54% of cases condoms were recommended, and information was given about emergency contraceptive methods. In 30%, combined, low-dose oral contraceptives were prescribed. However, in order to evaluate the use of contraceptives among adolescents more detailed studies are needed.

71

Adolescents have to buy prescribed contraceptives at full price, since there are no discounts for young people. The Latvian Association of Obstetricians and Gynecologists has turned to the government to find a way to finance contraceptives for teenagers and has explained the benefits this may bring to the future health of the population. However, this has not come about as yet, due to the economic situation in the country and the budget deficit.

Sex education

Sex education plays a very important role in the postponement of sexual involvement, in decreasing the number of unintended adolescent pregnancies, and in lowering the rate of STDs (Dexeus, 1996). While the increasing rates of pregnancy and STDs among young women indicate the necessity for education targeted at girls and boys, sex education is in fact needed for all age groups in Latvia. There have been some well coordinated efforts to improve sex education in Latvia for the benefit of young people. "Health promotion" activities have become increasingly popular. Sex education has not been incorporated yet into the school curriculum. It has been taught in approximately 250 schools on a voluntary basis (there are 1000 schools in Latvia). More than 600 teachers have sought training to become health education teachers in different institutions, but a unified program for teachers does not exist in Latvia, nor is there an accepted teaching program for all years.

The task of providing information, education, and communication is carried out by the nongovernmental organizations, such as Latvia's Association for Family Planning and Sexual Health and the Health Education Teacher Association.

The Youth Health Center, which was organized in February 1993, has been attended by 20 000 young people in order to get more information about their reproductive system, their health, contraception, sexuality, and other topics (Busa, 1996).

In Estonia sex education is part of the health education program included in the curricula of the fourth, seventh and tenth classes. Health education lessons are conducted by teachers of various specialties, by health workers, and by psychologists. The treatment of family planning and sex life in schools is often unsatisfactory due to the lack of suitable teaching materials and/or insufficient training of teachers. In this respect, the situation in Latvia is the same as in Estonia.

In Lithuania the Catholic Church has a strong influence on the government, especially on the ministers of education and health care. This influence interferes with the introduction of a family planning program and also sex education. This is, as it were, to "save life and moral values of society."

Heath care services for adolescents

The Youth Health Center in Riga is the only medical institution in Latvia that specializes in the provision of medical services for adolescents. Teenagers may have consultations with a gynecologist, a urologist, and a psychologist. In other outpatient clinics children below 18 pay a reduced fee for a consultation (one-fifth of the usual fee). Unfortunately, the attitude of the gynecologist toward young people is not always welcoming and friendly—the specialist sometimes fails to provide a degree of privacy, which discourages adolescents to seek medical attention. Several new youth health centers are going to be organized in smaller towns in the near future.

Adolescent reproductive health research needs

All the above data show that not much research has been performed to evaluate the reproductive health of adolescents in Eastern Europe. Statistical data are not available or are difficult to compare because standard definitions are not used in every country. The results of the research ought to be the source of reliable information that could be used to find the correct and the most cost-effective ways to solve the problem. These results should be the basis for national long-term programs to improve the reproductive health of adolescents in Eastern Europe.

Conclusions

The political and economic situation in Latvia and other Eastern European countries has a considerable influence on the role and lifestyle of young people in society. The main obstacles to improving the reproductive health of adolescents are as follows:

1. a low level of education, including sex education;
2. a carefree attitude among young people toward sexual relations and their own health;
3. an increase in the number of teenage prostitutes;
4. low use of modern contraceptives among teenagers;
5. a great number of unwanted pregnancies among teenage girls, which mostly end in induced abortions;
6. a high rate of STDs in the population.

A lot of work has been performed by nongovernmental organizations in order to improve the situation. They mostly rely on the support of international organizations in providing, for instance, a hot-line for teenagers in Latvia's Association for Family Planning and Sexual Health, a special leaflet on contraception for schoolchildren, lectures in schools, and activities in the cities. However, there is a need for greater support from the political decision-makers in the government and for them to understand the significance of the reproductive health of adolescents in the solution of demographic problems in the future in most of the countries of Eastern Europe. It is necessary to:

1. increase the number of youth health centers that would provide up-to-date information on health, sexual relations, and contraception;

2. provide access to modern contraceptives for teenagers free of charge or at a low price;

3. provide free contraception for teenage girls after an abortion;

4. introduce sex education as a compulsory subject in schools;

5. provide free examination of adolescents for STDs including an examination before abortion;

6. provide free treatment of adolescents for STDs;

7. improve legislation on the involvement of teenagers in prostitution.

Close cooperation between the government and nongovernmental organizations will promote the reproductive health of adolescents in Eastern European countries.

References

Busa, I. 1996. Youth health center [in Latvian]. In *Abstract book of the 1st conference—medical and social aspects of pediatric and adolescent gynaecology in Latvia and East Europe,* Latvia, Jurmala: Latvian Association of Gynaecologists and Obstetricians.

Chenet, L. 1996. Teenage fertility in the European Union. *Entre Nous, The European Family Planning Magazine* 32: 6–7.

Dexeus, S. 1996. Risks and benefits for adolescent contraception. *European Journal of Contraception and Reproductive Health Care* 1: 99–100.

Fathalla, M. F., et al. 1990. Adolescent sexuality and pregnancy. In *Reproductive health, global issues.* eds. Fathalla, M. F., Rosenfield, A., Indriso, C., Sen, D. K., and Ratnam, S. S. FIGO 3: 100–21.

Health in Riga. 1996. Riga City Council Health Department, Stock Company "Rigas Slimokases."

Karlen, H., and Hagner, C. 1996. Commercial sexual exploitation of children in some Eastern European countries (Estonia, Latvia, Lithuania, Poland,

Romania, Russia, Hungary). In *The international campaign to end child prostitution in Asian tourism,* Bangkok.

Miltina, I., and Lazdane, G. 1996. Pregnancy and deliveries for teenagers [in Latvian]. In *Abstract book of the 1ˢᵗ conference—medical and social aspects of pediatric and adolescent gynaecology in Latvia and East Europe*, Latvia, Jurmala: Latvian Association of Gynaecologists and Obstetricians.

Republic of Latvia. 1996. Medical care for pregnant women and neonates [in Latvian]. Riga: Health Department, Ministry of Welfare, Republic of Latvia.

UN. 1995. *The programme of action of the International Conference on Population and Development, Cairo 1994.* New York: United Nations.

UNDP. 1995. *Latvia, human development report.* New York: United Nations Development Fund.

UNDP. 1996. *Latvia, human development report.* Riga: United Nations Development Fund Riga Office.

WHO Regional Office for Europe and United Nations Population Fund. 1995. *Family planning and reproductive health in CCEE/NIS.* Geneva: World Health Organization.

Zumente, M. 1996. Contraceptive choice of adolescents [in Latvian]. In *Abstract book of the 1ˢᵗ conference—medical and social aspects of pediatric and adolescent gynaecology in Latvia and East Europe,* Latvia, Jurmala: Latvian Association of Gynaecologists and Obstetricians.

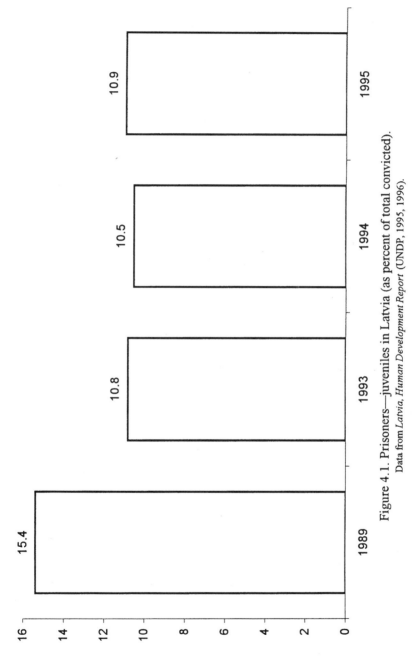

Figure 4.1. Prisoners—juveniles in Latvia (as percent of total convicted).
Data from *Latvia, Human Development Report* (UNDP, 1995, 1996).

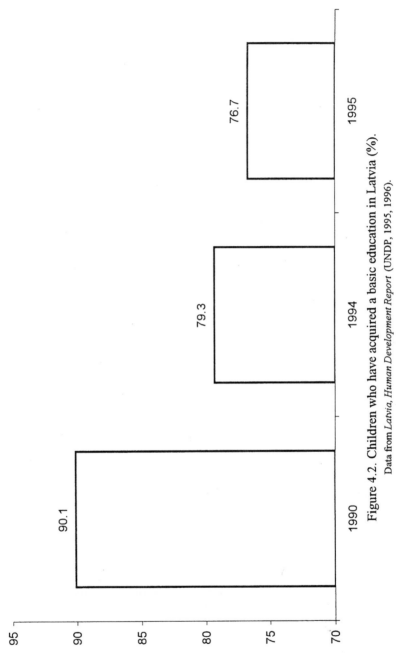

Figure 4.2. Children who have acquired a basic education in Latvia (%).
Data from *Latvia, Human Development Report* (UNDP, 1995, 1996).

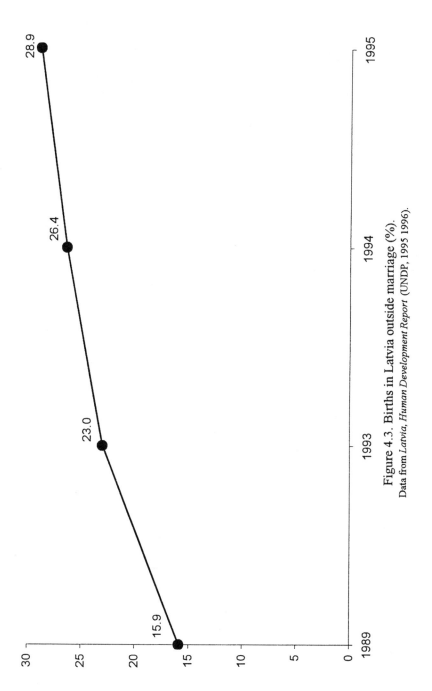

Figure 4.3. Births in Latvia outside marriage (%).
Data from *Latvia, Human Development Report* (UNDP, 1995 1996).

79

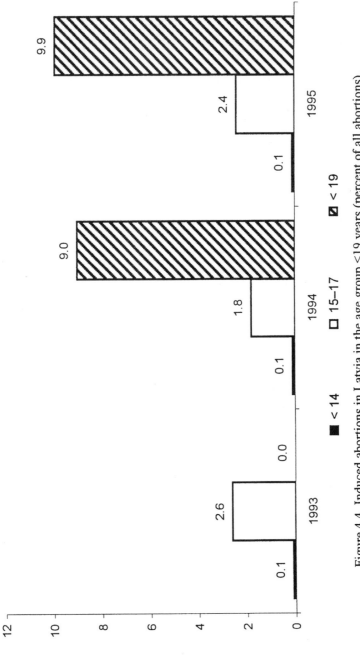

Figure 4.4. Induced abortions in Latvia in the age group <19 years (percent of all abortions).
Data from Bureau of Medical Statistics, Health Department, Ministry of Welfare, Republic of Latvia (1996).

■ < 14   □ 15–17   ▨ < 19

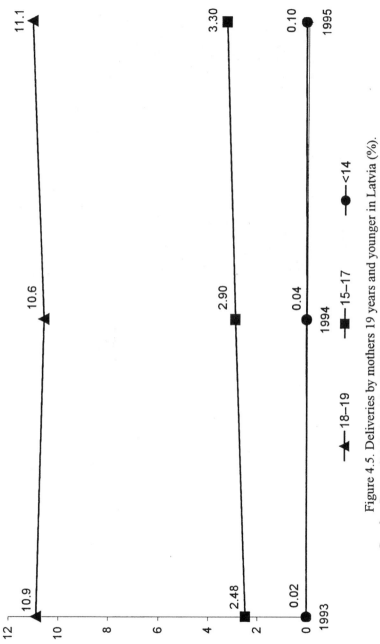

Figure 4.5. Deliveries by mothers 19 years and younger in Latvia (%).
Data from Bureau of Medical Statistics, Health Department, Ministry of Welfare, Republic of Latvia (1996).

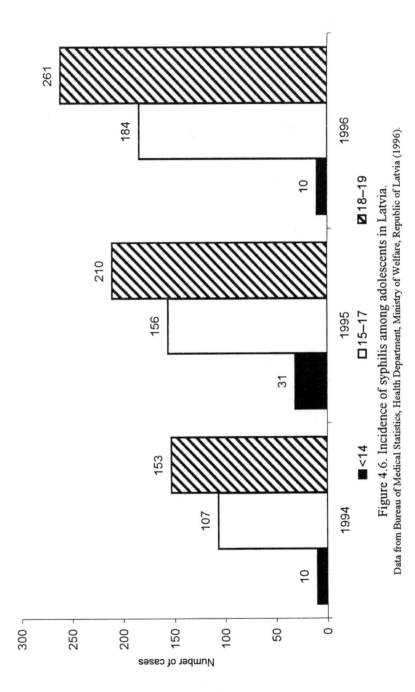

Figure 4.6. Incidence of syphilis among adolescents in Latvia.
Data from Bureau of Medical Statistics, Health Department, Ministry of Welfare, Republic of Latvia (1996).

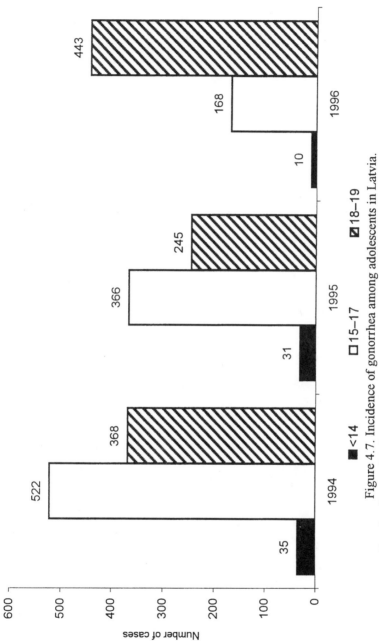

Figure 4.7. Incidence of gonorrhea among adolescents in Latvia.
Data from Bureau of Medical Statistics, Health Department, Ministry of Welfare, Republic of Latvia (1996).

Contraception:
current use and future perspectives

LÁSZLÓ KOVÁCS

Albert Szent-Györgyi Medical University, Department of Obstetrics and Gynaecology
WHO Collaborating Center for Research in Human Reproduction, Szeged, Hungary

Abstract

The current use of fertility regulating methods in the Eastern European countries is reviewed. The characteristic feature is the low prevalence of contraception and the high prevalence of termination of pregnancy, although there are major differences between the different countries. The health systems in the region are outlined in order to find an explanation for this unacceptable situation and to promote efforts to achieve changes. The statistical data convincingly point to the correlation of contraceptive prevalence and indicators of reproductive health. The impact of legislation on the use of fertility regulating methods is discussed. Action is suggested for an effective move from abortion to contraception.

Introduction

The area to be covered in this paper comprises the region of the former socialist or communist countries situated behind the one-time Iron Curtain, including the countries of the former Soviet Union, its former European satellites, and the former Yugoslavia. These countries have a number of common characteristics, but there are also numerous differences in their conditions that influence the status of general health and health policy, including the situation of obstetrics and gynecology and reproductive health. Most of these countries are currently undergoing economic transition; some of them are categorized as developing countries.

Contraception is one of the fields of reproductive health that has changed substantially during the past decade and many problems are still not solved. In Europe there are marked differences between the Western and Eastern halves. Induced abortion is still one of the major problems in the Eastern half, the prevalence of contraception is low, and frequently repeated abortion appears to many to be the only solution.

Background: reasons for current situation

It is common knowledge that the socialist–communist system in Europe collapsed some six to seven years ago. The standards in the various countries at that time differed somewhat, in part because the different dictatorial governments had ruled for different periods: for about 70 years in the former Soviet Union, and for "only" about 40 years in the satellites on its western flanks. The history and the standards of medicine in general, and of obstetrics and gynecology in particular, had also differed significantly from country to country in the region before the start of communist rule, and this is still apparent in the present status of family planning and reproductive health (Kovács, 1994).

One of the characteristic features of the current economic transition is that the state-controlled health system is changing back to the formerly mixed system, which includes both public and private services. The privatization of outpatient care centers is already underway in most of these countries, and the route toward the privatization of some public hospitals and larger centers has been prepared. However, the course of this privatization is proving chaotic, and the legal and organizational aspects are mostly highly inadequate. The insurance system is demonstrating growing pains in practically all of these countries, and there is usually only one health insurance company in each, with all the disadvantages of a monopoly.

The health services are either not financed on or are only partly financed on a fee-for-service basis, but usually receive standard support, irrespective of the quality and quantity of their activities. Correction of this ineffective system has begun, but it is far from perfect yet in most of these countries.

The salaries and incomes of health service employees, from doctors to assistant nurses, are very low, with a consequent low attraction for working in the health services, including a lack of staff and a high turnover, particularly among paramedical staff.

Overall, the standard of equipment, training, and medical technology in the former period was much lower in these countries than in Western Europe. However, there were great differences from country to country; some could maintain traditional contacts with the Western community, and in almost all of these countries there existed a few centers of excellence, partly to serve the political élite, but partly due to their very high-level scientific and clinical achievements and their active relations with Western partners. The average standard of obstetrics and gynecology was poor, and this is reflected in the health statistics and reproductive health indicators.

Family planning services are usually of a low level and information and education relating to family planning is lacking. Women are poorly informed about contraceptive use and are largely unaware of the long-term noncontraceptive benefits. Contraceptive methods, mainly hormonal, are refused because of the fear of complications. In most countries, abortion was approved as a method of birth control earlier than reliable contraception. Because of poor patient education and counseling, it is difficult to change the attitude of the population, and this is one of the main reasons for the low contraceptive prevalence and poor compliance.

Contraceptive use

It is almost impossible to assess the realistic situation of contraceptive prevalence and the ratio of reliable and less effective methods in this region. There have been a number of more or less professionally acceptable data collections and analyses. The published data are generally based on questionnaires, marketing data, and extrapolations of information on small groups. The overall data are usually not highly informative, as indicated in table 5.1, compiled from the data of a UN publication (United Nations, 1994). Meaningful comparisons of the prevalence data are virtually impossible because of the proportions of the reliable and unreliable methods (e.g. in Bulgaria: total prevalence 76%, with 2% of oral contraceptive use versus 69% of "nonsupply" methods).

The data collected in 1993 indicated that the overall use of contraceptives in the region was generally low: although it varied from 10% (Romania) to 92% (Slovenia) in 9 of the 16 countries, with populations totaling approximately 300 million people, the overall prevalence of contraceptive use was below 40% (Kovács, 1995). Similar, although somewhat different, rates for 1992–94 were published by WHO (WHO and UN Population Fund, 1995) (fig. 5.1).

Data relating to the use of different contraceptive methods are most complete for oral contraceptives and intrauterine devices (IUDs) (Kovács, 1995). The average use of oral contraceptives is 11.93%. In 8 countries the ratio of users is less than 10%, in 6 countries it is between 10 and 30%, and in 1 it is above 30% (fig. 5.2). The average use of IUDs is 13%. In 4 countries it is less than 10%, in 9 countries it is 10–20%, and in 2 countries it is above 20% (fig. 5.3).

It is important to emphasize, however, that in several countries neither oral contraceptives nor IUDs are available in sufficient quantity, nor is provision made for the continuity of supplies.

In most Eastern European countries there is no production of contraceptives, and any local products are generally less modern than the imported ones. Moreover, the more up-to-date imported products are more expensive than the domestic products. Again, in most countries contraceptives are provided at full price with no support from the health insurance system. This situation creates a serious inequity, because most women cannot afford up-to-date contraceptives, and adolescents and unemployed women with no income cannot afford contraceptives at all.

It is worth mentioning that access to abortion is usually cheaper than contraception in most of these countries. While abortion is performed free of charge for the lower income categories, the full price has to be paid for contraceptives even by the poorest, e.g., by adolescents who have no income.

The same conclusion was drawn in a publication of the WHO Regional Office for Europe. While contraceptive prevalence rates range from about 60 to 70% in some countries of Western Europe, they are less than 5% in some of the Eastern European countries. In many countries, the financial resources or the political will to make the necessary changes are lacking (WHO and UN Population Fund, 1995).

Although most of the Eastern European countries report a growing interest in contraceptives, limited availability and cost remove them as viable options for many people. Receiving an abortion for very little money, or even free, but having to give one-third of one's income for contraceptives rules out choice (WHO and UN Population Fund, 1995).

The Romanian situation, summarized in 1996 by Johnson, Horga, and Andronache, is characteristic of the region. In Romania modern contraceptive methods have not been readily available in the past and abortion has long been the primary form of fertility regulation. Although abortion was cheaper and more accessible than contraceptives in the period 1990–92, the costs and accessibility of abortion and contraception are currently similar. The real costs of an abortion includes a government fee (3000 lei, or less than $3 at December 1993), plus (as is commonly the case) the cost of a gift for the gynecologist, the attending nurse(s), and occasionally even the nurse who admits the woman to the hospital. By contrast, the cost of an IUD is in the range of 2000–3000 lei. The price of oral contraceptives ranges from 400 lei per cycle at an SECS Clinic (clinics run by the Society for Education on Contraception and Sexuality and funded by the United States Agency for International Development) to up to 5000 lei in some private pharmacies. There is no local manufacture of IUDs or oral contraceptives, although locally made condoms and spermicides synthesized by local pharmacists are available.

To increase the short-term use of modern contraception, public health priorities should be focused on the provision of a broad range of dependably available, low-cost, high-quality contraceptives distributed through a wide network of comprehensive family planning services staffed by well-trained providers. In addition, women who receive abortions on request should be provided with contraceptive counseling and methods to reduce the rate of repeated induced abortions.

Surgical contraception is very uncommon in Eastern Europe. The annual number of female sterilizations in the whole region is probably not more than several ten thousands, and the number of male sterilizations is 10 or 15 times less. A survey by Belaiche in 1994 showed that female sterilization for nonmedical but contraceptive indications was approved in only 3 of 7 Eastern European countries. Laparoscopy was used only in the same 3 countries, while sterilization for medical indications was performed by laparotomy in the other 4 countries. Male sterilization in 1994 was legally approved in 1 country (table 5.2).

Concerning the consequences, it is worth emphasizing that a statistical survey in the Eastern European countries clearly revealed a strong correlation between contraceptive prevalence and reproductive health indicators. In countries with a contraceptive prevalence below 40%, maternal mortality was as high as 28.5 per 100 000, infant mortality was 16.7 per 1000, and perinatal mortality was 15.4 per 1000. By comparison, in the countries with a contraceptive prevalence of 70% or more, maternal mortality was 12.8 per 100 000, while infant mortality was 7.9 and perinatal mortality was 8.6 per 1000 (table 5.3) (Kovács, 1995).

The impact of legislation

Legislation also influences contraception. The use of surgical contraception is minimal in this region. As compared with developing countries, where its prevalence is 45.3% of contraceptive users (it is 14.2% in developed countries), the several ten thousand reported sterilizations are negligible. The reasons are different in the different countries. In most countries, surgical contraception is not approved legally, but it is nevertheless performed by some doctors. In such cases, of course, they are not covered by their professional insurance.

In countries such as Hungary, where surgical contraception is legal, a limiting factor is that the health insurance scheme does not reimburse the expenses. Surgical contraception for other than medical indications is provided at full cost and is expensive: more than one month's income on average.

Family planning services only partly fall under the health insurance system. Several assisted reproductive treatments are covered with limitations, and are likewise expensive, creating a situation of inequity for the poor infertile couple.

Conclusions

The need and the possibilities for better future perspectives are outlined in the conclusions of The Szeged Declaration (1994). The major problems identified were the low level or lack of training of professionals, deficiencies in knowledge of current family planning methods among professionals, consumers, policymakers, and media representatives, the lack of supplies of modern contraceptives to meet the needs of the population, the lack of sex education in schools, and the high level of induced abortions.

In the majority of the countries in this region, there is a need for the establishment of a system for the delivery of high quality family planning services. This imposes a requirement for the establishment of a system for a continuous supply of contraceptives through national family planning programs, by government and/or nongovernmental organizations.

To increase contraceptive use, countries in this region should consider the establishment of extensive educational programs on current family planning methods and other aspects of reproductive health for their health professionals, consumers, and representatives of the media. Sex education in schools should be encouraged. Governments should be encouraged to invest more in setting up and running family planning services and programs.

It may be worth mentioning that in 1990 the yearly per capita health expenditure in the 16 countries varied from $26 (Albania) to $185 (Hungary). For comparison, the yearly per capita health expenditure for the 5.5 billion people of the world was $323 (World Bank, 1993).

References

Belaiche, R. 1994. Human sterilisation. *Syngof* 18: 31–5.

Johnson, B. R., Horga, M., and Andronache, L. 1996. Women's perspectives on abortion in Romania. *Social Science and Medicine* 42: 521–30.

Kovács, L. 1994. The current situation of obstetrics and gynaecology in Central and Eastern Europe. *Journal of the Canadian Society of Obstetrics and Gynecology* 16: 2166–71.

Kovács, L. 1995. Political and social influences on women's choices of fertility regulation. In *From contraception to reproductive health care,* ed. M. Elstein, 89–106. London and New York: Parthenon.

United Nations. 1994. World contraceptive use 1994 (ST, ESA, SER.A) 143. New York: UN.

The Szeged Declaration. 1994. Assessment of research and service needs on reproductive health in Eastern Europe—concerns and commitments. *Human Reproduction* 9: 750–2.

WHO Regional Office for Europe and United Nations Population Fund. 1995. Family planning and reproductive health in CCEE/NIS. Doc. EUR/ICP/FMLY 94 03/PB01. Copenhagen: World Health Organization.

World Bank. 1993. *World development report—investing in health.* Oxford: Oxford University.

Table 5.1

Contraceptive use in several countries. Extracted from *World Contraceptive Use*

(United Nations, 1994)

Country	Year	Age range years	Users (%)	Steriliza- tion male (%)	Sterilization female (%)	Pill (%)	IUD (%)	Condom (%)	Other supply method (%)	Nonsupply method (%)
Bulgaria	1976	18–44	76	1	1	2	2	2	–	69
Czech Republic	1993	15–44	69	3	–	8	15	19	0.2	24
Hungary	1988	15–39	73	–	–	39	19	4	1	11
Poland	1977	<45	75	–	–	7	2	14	3	49
Romania	1993	15–44	57	1	–	3	4	4	2	43
Slovakia	1991	15–44	74	4	–	5	11	21	–	32
Yugoslavia (former)	1976	<45	55	–	–	5	2	2	3	43

Table 5.2

Survey on human sterilization in Eastern Europe (Belaiche, 1994)

Country	Contraceptive	Medical	Female	Laparoscopy	Vasectomy
Bulgaria	−	+	−	−	−
Georgia	+	+	+	+	−
Hungary	+	+	+	+	+
Lithuania	−	+	−	−	−
Poland	−	+	−	−	−
Romania	−	+	−	−	−
Slovakia	+	+	+	+	−

Table 5.3

Contraceptive prevalence and reproductive health indicators (Kovács, 1995)

	Contraceptive prevalence		
	< 40	40–70	> 70
No. of countries	9	4	2
No. of abortions	5 712 100	306 980	66 257
Women aged 15–49 years	70 319 120	6 701 907	2 479 506
Percentage of abortions	8	5	3
Maternal mortality (per 100 000)	28.5	8.2	12.8
Infant mortality (per 1000)	16.7	9.4	7.9
Perinatal mortality (per 1000)	15.4	11.5	8.6

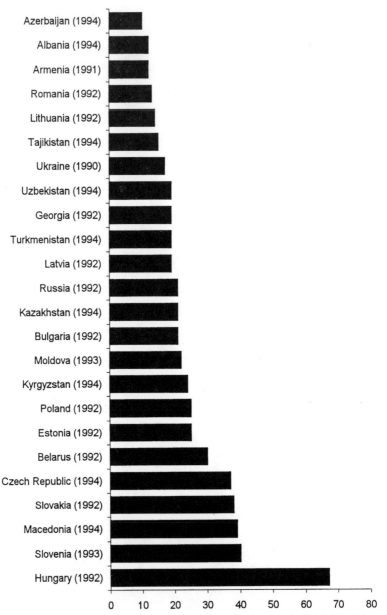

Figure 5.1. Contraceptive prevalence rate (effective methods) 1992–94.
Source: WHO and UN Population Fund (1995).

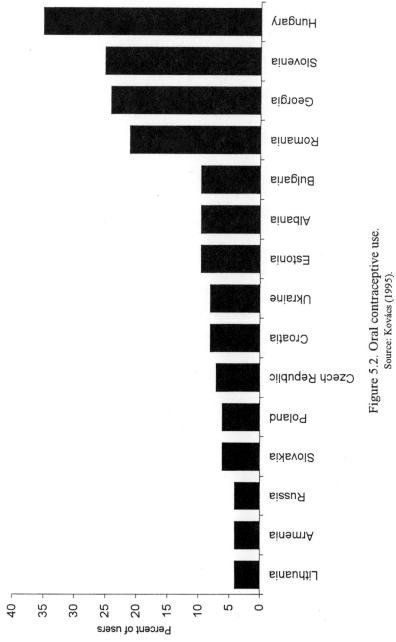

Figure 5.2. Oral contraceptive use.
Source: Kovács (1995).

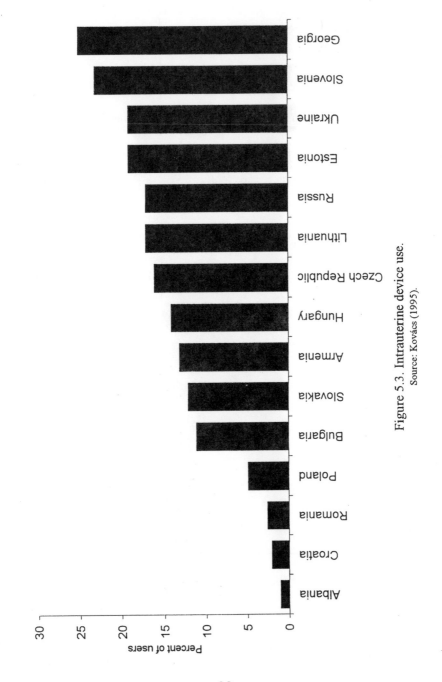

Figure 5.3. Intrauterine device use.
Source: Kovács (1995).

How can the rates
of induced abortion be reduced?

MIHAI HORGA[1] and FRANK LÜDICKE[2]

[1] Center of Public Health, Targu-Mures, Romania
[2] Clinic for Infertility and Gynaecological Endocrinology, University Hospital,
Geneva, Switzerland

Abstract

The magnitude and multitude of reproductive health implications
make abortion a major public health issue for the countries of
Eastern Europe and the Newly Independent States. The objective
of this paper is to outline the current extent of the abortion issue
in this region, to attempt to identify the factors leading to this
situation, and to suggest possible solutions. The motivation to reduce abortion rates and the process that leads women throughout
this region to resort to this method of regulating fertility are
investigated in order to find efficient strategies to decrease the
rates of abortion. Several preventive strategies to bring down the
number of abortions are described, intervening in one or more of
the following three areas: socioeconomic, behavioral change, and
health. The objective of all these strategies should be to prevent
the need for abortion, and the underlying mechanism should be
the development of preventive thinking instead of a curative one.
Solutions for reducing abortion rates are only partially medical,
they are mostly economic, social, and educational. Countries in
the region must shift from "post-factum" to preventive family
planning strategies, from an "abortion culture" to a "contraception
culture." Preventing unwanted pregnancies through the provision
of information, and education and access to modern contraceptive

methods represents the most effective strategy for decreasing the induced abortion rates. Abortion must not be promoted as a method of fertility regulation, but it should be recognized as an important component of reproductive health.

Introduction

The practice of abortion is a worldwide phenomenon, and, as one of the oldest and most widely used methods of fertility regulation, it will always occur because unwanted pregnancies will always appear. Abortion is also an emotionally charged issue that has always produced ideological, ethical, religious, political, and juridical debates among various groups of professionals and the general public.

From an individual perspective, termination of an unwanted pregnancy is the result of a personal decision. Women who wish to avoid an unwanted pregnancy have three options: abstinence, effective contraception, or abortion. There is a great difference between a wanted pregnancy, with the joy and fulfillment it brings, and an unwanted pregnancy, with the desperation and rejection that can accompany it. Confronted with an unwanted pregnancy, women may choose to terminate it regardless of their socioeconomic or cultural background, legal codes, religious sanctions, or the risk to physical or mental well-being. The decision to terminate a pregnancy can create psychological stress, and the abortion experience itself may be traumatic for a woman, especially if she is young and pregnant for the first time, or if the abortion experience represents her first contact with the medical system. Taken together, the circumstances surrounding an unwanted pregnancy and the decision to have an abortion are important milestones in a woman's reproductive life.

From a social perspective, abortion represents a major public health issue that is especially unfortunate because it is almost entirely preventable. For Eastern Europe, abortion represents a particularly important problem, given its magnitude.

The objectives of this paper are to outline the current extent of the abortion issue in Eastern Europe, to attempt to identify the factors that contribute to this, and to suggest possible interventions that might help reduce the incidence of abortion. The term Eastern Europe (EE) used throughout this paper includes 27 countries with economies in transition that have similar economic, social, and political characteristics and are localized geographically in five subregions: Eastern Europe, the Baltic states, Commonwealth of Independent States, Central Asian Republics and Kazakhstan, and the former Yugoslavia (WHO and UN Population Fund, 1995).

What is the magnitude of the abortion issue in EE ?

The 1993 WHO estimates for the worldwide incidence of abortion were 19 900 000 cases. These abortions have led to 67 000 maternal deaths and have affected the health of 4 800 000 women (WHO 1995b).

In the 27 countries of EE there are 627 million inhabitants with a wide diversity of cultural backgrounds. However, the effects of the political and economic transition and ongoing reforms confer a similar profile to these former communist countries in terms of general trends and reproductive health problems. Table 6.1 lists the prevalence rates for fertility, birth, abortion, and contraception in these countries.

One outstanding characteristic of the countries in this region is the extremely high use of abortion, together with a low contraceptive use (WHO and UN Population Fund, 1995). Abortion rates in these countries are very high, in some cases equaling or even exceeding the birthrate by two or three times. The rates range from 14 abortions per 1000 women in Poland to 239 abortions per 1000

101

women in Azerbaijan, while Western Europe countries have rates below 20 per 1000 women.

These rates must be interpreted with care, since official health statistics in these countries are sometimes dated, and different definitions from internationally accepted ones may have been used. Also, the number of abortions performed in the emerging private medical sector may not always be adequately reported. Even if they are not distorted by underreporting, these figures indicate that, for EE countries, abortion represents the principal means of fertility regulation.

Although sharing the same continent, a different historical and political evolution has led to a gap between the countries of Eastern and Western Europe in terms of most health indicators. While many general health indicators are similar to those in Western European countries, reproductive health indicators are very different (WHO and Population Fund, 1995). This situation has several historical and political explanations.

Abortion has been a common and widespread form of fertility regulation throughout the formerly communist countries of EE (Frejka, 1983), being legalized in most of these countries after the Soviet model from 1920, aiming at creating conditions for a new communist society and designed to recognize the equal status of women (David, 1992). The fact that modern contraceptive methods had not yet been developed favored the establishment of induced abortion as the main method of fertility regulation.

Around 1956–57, again following the Soviet example, most EE countries (with the exception of Yugoslavia, the German Democratic Republic, and Albania) promoted laws permitting abortion on broad grounds. The Soviet model of birth control that promoted abortion instead of contraception was characterized by broad legal grounds for abortion, low use of modern contraceptive methods, and a lack of contraceptive information and services (Popov, 1993). This policy led to an extremely high abortion rate and had long lasting consequences on women's and men's attitudes and practices until today.

When the fertility rates in these countries fell below the replacement level, one of the measures taken by some communist regimes (Romania, Bulgaria, Czechoslovakia, Hungary) was to ban abortion and contraception, along with providing incentives for child-bearing (Frejka, 1983). That pro-natalist policy had a negative impact on women's reproductive health, as the Romanian experience has sadly demonstrated with a huge increase in maternal mortality and morbidity, and only re-enforced the use of abortion (this time illegal) for avoiding unwanted births. The lack of sex and contraceptive education and low contraceptive availability and use that accompanied this policy had a profound impact that still persists nearly ten years after the fall of communism at the end of the 1980s.

Why should abortion rates be reduced ?

The motivation to reduce abortion rates may be connected to individual and social factors, among which abortion-related mortality and morbidity, the impact on women's future fertility, the cost to society, and concern about population decline are often mentioned. Abortion contributes to maternal mortality and represents an important cause of morbidity among women of reproductive age in EE countries. Recent statistics show that mortality rates from abortion-related causes ranges between 2 and 34 deaths per 100 000 livebirths for EE countries, while in most Western European countries the figure is lower than 2 (WHO, 1993).

Abortion-related morbidity is more difficult to assess. Short-term complications (like trauma, hemorrhage, and pelvic infection) and late complications (like cervical and uterine adhesions and secondary infertility) are described. They may have an impact on reproductive life and later pregnancies (Hogue, 1986; Atrash, and Hogue, 1990, Grebsheva, 1992, Serbanescu et al., 1995). Maternal morbidity after induced abortion can cause long-term disability or even partial invalidity (WHO and Population Fund, 1995). The psychological impact of abortion and its possible complications have been also documented (Spinelli et al., 1993, Holmgren, and Uddenberg, 1994).

Information is scare on the consequences of induced abortion in EE, in terms of reproductive morbidity and the costs involved. The assumption that abortion on request has no implications for the future ability to conceive is mainly based on existing studies performed in Western countries, where abortion is performed under different conditions (Hogue, 1986; Benson Gold, 1990). This has not yet been documented for EE, and available (mostly anecdotal) information suggests that impaired fertility after induced abortion is more frequent, given the high number of procedures that have to be performed under limitations of time and resources. More research is needed, however, to document the specific situation in EE countries. Although abortion is legal in these countries, it is the quality of the abortion services that ultimately affects its safety. We believe that the long-term effects of the millions of abortions being performed in the region will become apparent only in the coming years, possibly creating a crisis in reproductive health and especially infertility services.

Other reasons for reducing the abortion rates are related to social factors. The question of the price paid by society for abortion has several aspects. The great number of abortion procedures performed is placing a burden on the public health system; if complications occur, the costs rise significantly. For instance, the management of an incomplete abortion, which often results from an illegal abortion, has been shown to use up a large proportion of the budgets of obstetric and gynecology departments (Liskin, 1980; Johnson et al., 1993a).

There is also concern about the decline in fertility to rates below replacement levels in countries of the region. According to the

United Nations World Population Prospects (medium variant projection), the population of EE will decrease from 309 288 000 in 1994 to 299 374 000 in 2025 (UN, 1995b). Fertility in EE has already declined from 2.1 children per woman during 1980–85 to 1.6 children per woman during 1990–95 (Shah, 1996). Between 1990 and 1995 there was a negative population growth rate (–0.1%), compared to the period between 1980 and 1985 (+0.6%) (UN, 1995b). This trend is not uniform, with the populations of Hungary and Bulgaria, for example, declining by about 2.5%, while the populations of Poland and Slovakia continue to grow. Reasons for this situation are common to all of these countries and include sharp declines in fertility, rising or stagnant mortality, and out-migration.

What becomes apparent from these figures is that there seems to be a desire for fewer children and smaller families in the EE countries. The assumption (used sometimes to promote restrictive abortion laws) that this trend in fertility is induced or maintained by a high utilization of abortion is not accurate. The societies in transition from a centrally planned economy to a market economy are facing new, challenging problems arising from this transition. Economic hardships, unemployment (affecting women as well as men), inequalities in income and rising poverty have led to less desire to conceive, which is the main reason for the decline in fertility.

The magnitude of the phenomenon and the multitude of implications for reproductive health make abortion a major public health issue for EE countries. Reducing abortion rates through various available strategies should, therefore, be a priority for the governments in the region and for international agencies.

What are the factors that lead to abortion ?

In order to find viable and efficient strategies to decrease the rates of abortion, it is necessary to understand the process that leads women throughout EE to resort to this method of fertility regulation. The question has a particular relevance since substantial funds have been allocated to build and develop family planning services in these countries and to import modern contraceptives. Still, prevalence rates for modern contraception remain low, abortion remains the main method of fertility regulation, and little is known about the decision process that leads a woman to abortion.

This process begins when a pregnancy is considered unwanted or mistimed by the woman and/or her partner. It is estimated that, overall, half of the pregnancies are unplanned, and a quarter are certainly unwanted (UNDP/UNFPA/WHO/World Bank Special Programme of Research, Development and Research Training in Human Reproduction, 1994). It is evident that the decision to conceive or not and the right time for a pregnancy are influenced by many factors, among which socioeconomic and cultural ones are predominant. The leading reasons (stated by almost two-thirds of the respondents) for having an induced abortion in the 1993 Czech Republic Reproductive Health Survey were the desire to have no more children (34%) or to wait longer for a child (15%), or the inability to afford another child (14%) (Czech Statistical Office, 1995). The 1993 Romanian Reproductive Health Survey showed that 67% of abortions were performed to limit or space children and 20% for economic or social reasons (low income, crowding, fear of losing a job) (IOMC and CDC, 1995).

No matter what the initial reason for not wanting a pregnancy (which is rarely a medical issue), one must examine the process that leads to the occurrence of unwanted or unplanned pregnancies in order to find effective solutions (fig. 6.1). There are no major legal barriers and all these countries have initiated and developed family planning programs that offer at least the basic modern contraceptives. Still, as shown before, there is an unusually high incidence of abortion despite contraceptives being available.

A sexually active woman who wishes to avoid a pregnancy has two options: abstinence or contraception. For those who use contraception, failure of the contraceptive method is one of the factors involved. The use of traditional methods, associated with high failure rates, and inconsistent or incorrect use of modern methods are responsible for some of these pregnancies.

Data from the Romanian Reproductive Survey show that, overall, one in four women became pregnant while using a contraceptive method. The rate is understandably higher (30%) for traditional methods. Explanations for modern contraceptive failure include improper use, but there is also a possibility of poor quality contraceptives obtained from uncontrolled sources.

For many of these countries, especially for those with a long history of banned contraceptives, nonuse of contraception (in the form of either no contraception or no modern contraception) is the key factor that leads to unwanted pregnancies. Contraceptive use in the region is low overall, with contraceptive prevalence rates generally under 40%. Rates range from 7 (in Azerbaijan) to 62% (in Hungary), and there is a heavy reliance on traditional methods needing no supply (UN, 1994b; UNFPA, 1995). Understanding the reasons why women and men reject modern contraception methods is of utmost importance for designing preventive strategies and for avoiding the waste of funds.

Available studies show that a small percentage of women do not use modern contraception because they do not know about it (Sahatci, 1993b; Bruyniks, 1994; IOMC and CDC, 1995). This reveals one of the most devastating, long-term effects of the prohibition imposed by the communist regimes: the lack of knowledge about contraception that is present to different extents in all factors that lead to abortion. This lack of information is found among women and men of reproductive age, but it is even more important in older ages, where it might be extremely difficult to reverse after a lifetime of traditional sexual practices.

Of those women who know, some do not want to use modern contraception. This attitude may be due to a mistaken evaluation of the reproductive goals of the couple or of the health status of the woman. In a few cases, a planned pregnancy suddenly becomes unwanted because of a change in life circumstances. These cases are almost impossible to prevent. But in most cases, women believe they cannot become pregnant because they are protected by various factors and they do not know that they should use an effective method. The trust in the natural method of withdrawal and partner protection is responsible for an overwhelming number of cases. Moreover, cases where they do not have a stable relationship, have divorced or are separated from the partner, do not have frequent intercourse, or do not anticipate having unprotected intercourse result in unwanted pregnancies. In the absence of appropriate information, breastfeeding may be also considered an effective method. Also, after having tried unsuccessfully to become pregnant, some women believe that they are infertile and therefore take no protective measures. These cases also reflect a lack of appropriate knowledge about the efficacy of different methods of pregnancy prevention.

Some cases of contraceptive nonuse represent a deliberate rejection, motivated by a variety of reasons, such as lack of trust in the effectiveness and real protection of modern contraceptives, fear of the complications they could produce (either based on problems encountered in the past using a modern contraceptive method, or on misinformation about the side effects of modern contraceptives, particularly hormonal contraception and intrauterine devices). Without adequate information, some women find modern contraceptives difficult or inconvenient to use. Traditional views on sex make some women feel embarrassed to use them and promote use of a traditional method. In the same context, modern contraceptive use is sometimes associated with promiscuous sexual behavior (UNFPA, 1995). Although some religions may forbid the use of contraception, that has been shown to play an unimportant role in EE (Ketting et al., 1992; Johnson et al., 1996). On the contrary, one can see in these countries sociocultural norms that make the use of abortion as a method of regulating fertility acceptable, since it has been practiced for generations. It is interesting to note that the right to abortion granted to women in this transition period was assumed to be an essential ingredient of modern democratic practice (Kligman, 1992), and freedom of reproductive choice has sometimes been interpreted as freedom to have an induced abortion. This complex combination of perceptions, beliefs, attitudes, and practices, whose roots may be found in the historical and cultural background of the region, together make a true "abortion culture" that is extremely resistant to change.

The majority of these subjective factors result from a lack of knowledge about modern contraception, caused and maintained by the lack of correct information and circulation of incorrect information through different channels. The sources of this information may be the family, sexual partners, friends, or colleagues, but unfortunately they are also within the official educational health care, or media system. This aspect deserves a closer analysis.

For years, sex education was used to promote social control over individual behavior (Bostandjiev, 1992), and the task of teachers was to repress adolescent sexuality and maintain control over their sexual behavior. With such a background, and with no appropriate training, few educators dare to embark on the difficult task of teaching "uncomfortable" ideas related to sexuality and contraception.

Another aspect is the position of providers of a certain generation, who are opposed to prescribing modern contraception, or even favor abortion to the detriment of modern contraception, considering it safer (Jacobson, 1990; Johnson et al., 1993b; Visser et al., 1993b, 1993c, 1994). This attitude derives also from inadequate training and lack of continuing education on the indications and side effects of modern contraceptives and leads to all sorts of medical barriers. In Russia, it is thought that the main influence on public opinion about oral contraceptives is the negative attitude of Russian doctors (Popov et al., 1993). This attitude has historical explanations, since the Ministry of Public Health of the former USSR published in 1974 an instructive letter on the side effects and complications of oral contraceptives, reinforced by another document in 1983 that in fact sustained the prohibition of oral contraceptives for contraceptive purposes (Popov, 1993, Popov et al., 1993). Oral contraceptives have a surprisingly negative image also in the Czech Republic, which has a history of contraception use (Ketting et al., 1992).

Other reasons for not using modern contraception include restrictions on contraception use. Two main groups may be included in this category: the medical reasons and the partner's opposition. The medical barriers are closely related to the level of knowledge and professionalism in the provider community (Cottingham, and Mehta, 1993). Most current providers have received their education from outdated textbooks and facts that refer to the older generation of contraceptives (Johnson et al., 1993b; Visser et al., 1993b) and they continue to convey misperceptions about the contraindications and adverse effects of modern contraceptives.

The role of the male partner is also important in the decision whether to use contraception or to have an abortion. Often men consider contraception a woman's responsibility and refuse to be involved, and there are groups within the general population where men readily accept no contraceptive use. Since EE societies are traditionally male authoritarian societies, this might have an affect on the decision not to use contraception.

Access to family planning services and to modern contraceptive methods is also a major problem. The incidence of induced abortion was inversely correlated with access to and availability of safe, effective contraception (WHO and UN Population Fund, 1995). Although EE countries have inherited an extensive health care system, with many facilities and providers, historically this has developed as a hospital-based, curative system, and preventive health care, including family planning services, were not very well

110

understood until recently (UNFPA, 1995). Health care reform in these countries is also in the early stages, but the availability of contraceptives is limited and they are relatively high priced. In some countries, family planning is not included in the primary medical care package. In the absence of an adequate information and distribution system, many women do not know where to get modern contraceptives or cannot afford to buy them.

Besides the difficulties in accessing good quality contraceptives, easy access to a low cost, reasonably safe abortion may be viewed as a cause of its high incidence (Frejka, 1990). As long as it is cheaper to have an abortion than to obtain good quality contraceptives, and as long as women lack the necessary knowledge to choose between the two, they will continue to use the more familiar option of abortion (Johnson et al., 1993b).

The quality of the abortion services in EE leaves much to be desired. When abortion is performed in a setting of limited resources and a high caseload, as is the case in many of these countries, this may compromise the quality and safety of the medical produce, with possible health consequences. The method of sharp curettage is still used in many centers, alone or in conjunction with vacuum aspiration. Good information and counseling, which have been found useful to alleviate patients' fears, are often lacking, demonstrating an absence of understanding of and attention to women's motivations and needs (Leonard, and Ladipo, 1994).

Finally, even if none of the factors previously highlighted for not using contraception are present, some women do not use contraception and do not offer a satisfactory reason. Some of them might not have decided to use a modern contraceptive method, and even if they receive a prescription or contraception recommendation, still do not use it. The reasons behind this attitude are very complex and difficult to assess, but they seem to relate to either a wrong or an incomplete perception of the risks generated by an unsafe sexual practice.

Once an unwanted pregnancy has occurred, there are only two choices: abortion or birth. Facing this situation, few women agree to carry the pregnancy to term, and, unfortunately, abortion is the easiest way to manage the problem. Abortion is not restricted to young, unmarried women who cannot afford to have a child, but it is also used by married women to limit family size or postpone a birth in the absence of effective contraception (WHO, 1995a). Many women who have an abortion want to have a child later and the idea of giving the newborn up for adoption is not always acceptable, therefore abortion emerges as the choice.

How can abortion rates be decreased?

Having reviewed the factors that lead to high abortion rates, several strategies appear as possible preventive interventions to reduce the number of abortions (fig. 6.2). These strategies fall under one or more of three areas of intervention: socioeconomic, behavioral change, and health. The objective of all these strategies should be to prevent the need for abortion, not the abortion itself, and the underlying mechanism should be to develop preventive thinking instead of a curative one. One must start by understanding women's attitudes and behavior and attempt to change the "abortion culture" by providing accurate information, appropriate family planning services, and good supplies of contraceptives, while at the same time respecting their right to choose abortion.

The strategies and actions outlined in this chapter may be applied to all countries. However, they must be adjusted to specific national and local contexts in each EE country, taking into account their historic, demographic, cultural, socioeconomic, and economic characteristics. The result should be an environment in which women and men are able to exercise real choices in their reproductive lives.

A fundamental intervention that influences the desire to conceive is an improvement in socioeconomic conditions that will lead to fewer unwanted pregnancies and thus to possibly less need for abortion. Improvement in the status of women, and in their educational, economic, and social conditions, with more equal sharing in family and childbearing responsibilities, will lay the groundwork for achieving their reproductive goals. Moreover, improvements in both the status and reproductive health of women have many implications and benefits for the entire society (The Allen Guttmacher Institute, 1995).

Liberalizing rather than restricting the legal status of abortion is important, since controversy over, and even opposition to, abortion still exists in some EE countries. The new abortion laws in Poland and Hungary restrict the conditions under which a pregnancy can be terminated (Nowicka, 1993a, 1993b; Berbik, 1994). Abortion is undoubtedly a challenging political issue, and there is often little political interest in improving access to high-quality abortion services. There are even fears in some EE countries that abortion could be banned again (Chudikova, 1992).

Contrary to what legislators have sometimes intended, legally restricting of abortion does not necessarily lead to a marked decrease in the number of abortions (IPPF, 1989; Cook, 1993). The reproductive policies imposed in EE countries for more than forty years, with periods of liberalization alternating with periods of repression, clearly reveal that instead of reducing the number of abortions globally, repressive laws only increase the number of clandestine and unreported unsafe abortions. When a society restricts abortion through legislation, it only causes a shift from safe to unsafe abortions (Wolf, 1994). As the Romanian experience clearly demonstrated, the legal restriction of abortion is no solution, and the consequences may be dramatic in terms of increased maternal mortality and morbidity (Hord et al., 1991; Stephenson et al., 1992; David, and Baban, 1996). Moreover, a repressive policy has not been proven to have any durable impact whatsoever on the birthrate. Therefore, policymakers and health administrators must be convinced of the need to remove all barriers to a legal and safe abortion in law, in health regulations, and in clinical policies (Greenslade et al., 1993). However, as the ICPD Programme of Action states, any measures or changes related to abortion within the health system can only be determined at the national or local level according to the national legislative process (UN, 1995a).

But the most important component of these strategies is to spread knowledge about contraception through education, information, counseling, guidance, and support. Such information conveyed to women and men must include specific messages about pregnancy and abortion: information about missed periods, symptoms of pregnancy, pregnancy tests, what to do in case of suspected pregnancy, and where and how to have an abortion. Information should especially be targeted toward young people (to encourage responsible sexual behavior and delayed childbearing among adolescents) and women who are disadvantaged and who have a low level of education.

The channels through which these messages should be delivered include parents, educators, physicians, nurses, pharmacists, and the media. A perception seems to exist among women that family planning knowledge is controlled solely by gynecologists (Johnson et al., 1993b; Visser et al., 1993a), therefore the subjective value of information received from this source is high. This only stresses the importance of the type of messages conveyed by these professionals. Unfortunately, for many gynecologists, abortion is still the rule, and they do not seem interested, and have no time, to give information on family planning (Johnson et al., 1996). Among gynecologists there are still opinions that support the idea that a properly performed abortion has a lower risk of complication than contraception. Such attitudes demonstrate the need for better training and continued education of service providers in EE countries. Postgraduate courses and the integration of family planning

114

into the curriculum for medical students are two important measures (Visser et al., 1993c; Sahatci, 1993a). Still, authority-based medicine is the rule in EE, and evidence-based medicine, using modern scientific findings in clinical practice and training has still to be accepted and applied. In this aspect, the medical eligibility criteria for contraceptive use recently developed by WHO represent a powerful tool in removing these medical barriers to modern contraception and should be disseminated as widely as possible and incorporated into national guidelines and local practices.

Not only clients and providers, but also educators and media professionals in EE require education and information on family planning. The role of the media is particularly important, as it reaches vast audiences with information that may increase awareness of the behaviors that may put a woman at risk of an unwanted pregnancy.

Increasing male involvement in women's health issues may also help increase the use of modern contraceptives and subsequently contribute to reducing the abortion rates. Programs and services should include special components that address the role and responsibility of men in preventing unwanted pregnancies.

Increase access to contraception. One of the most efficient strategies shown to decrease abortion rates is to increase and broaden access to family planning services that offer efficient, modern contraceptives (Tbilisi Declaration, 1990). The relation between contraceptive use and abortion is complex, but there are many examples to substantiate this approach (Henshaw, and Morrow, 1990; Bruyniks, 1994; Djusubalieva, 1994). The issue of access has several dimensions that have to be addressed by these strategies. Availability of good quality contraceptives is definitely the most important, but it must be associated with affordability to the individual, which is affected by whether or not there are government subsidies. Promotion of modern contraceptive methods, through the media, through providers, and through other channels, can significantly increase access. As already mentioned, the attitudes and behavior of providers may especially influence the choice and use of contraceptive methods

Improvements in abortion services should include the safest methods of abortion and postabortion counseling and contraception to help prevent repeat unwanted pregnancies and abortion. Vacuum aspiration, recognized as the best method for early induced abortions, and treatment of incomplete abortion should become the standard procedure (Koontz, and Conly, 1993; Khomassuridze, 1994). Introducing modern technologies for abortion can improve a woman's access to safe, high-quality services, and reduce complications (Greenslade et al., 1993). The introduction of medical abortion services using anti-progestins and prostaglandins has been proposed as a way of expanding safe abortion services in the first trimester of pregnancy (WHO, 1994). Technological improvements in abortion services must be associated with the appropriate training of abortion care providers.

The appropriate technology and the technical competence of the providers are only part of the problem of quality of abortion care. The postabortion period offers a unique opportunity to help women find a solution to some of the problems that may have contributed to the unwanted pregnancy. Women usually have a legal or a clandestine induced abortion because they wish to avoid unwanted births but lack the necessary information or means to do that. Because the abortion procedure is performed in a gynecological service that often has few connections to a preventive family planning service, this important group of women is often neglected in terms of postabortion family planning (Wolf, and Benson, 1994). Approaching them with contraceptive counseling, information, and even supplying methods during this event might help avoid another abortion by breaking the cycle of unwanted pregnancy. Women need to know that they can become pregnant again before the next period, need to learn about modern contraceptive methods, and need to learn about how they can obtain them (Leonard, and Ladipo, 1994).

Counsel on other alternatives. A woman having an unwanted or unplanned pregnancy needs emotional support and help in order to make a decision about whether to have an abortion or not. The choice of adoption is not always at hand, and even if she accepts the idea, she must know how to proceed. Strategies to deal with these pregnancies must be developed and properly advertised in order to avoid termination of at least some unwanted pregnancies.

Research is an important component of any effort to stop the high rates of abortion. There are several lines of investigation with potential impact in this field. Research on contraceptive technology may lead to the development of more effective and reliable contraceptives, thus reducing the number of unwanted pregnancies and consequent abortions (Segal, and LaGuardia, 1990). Social science research into determinants of choice and use of fertility regulating methods is of paramount importance in helping to identify issues that cause individuals and couples to reject contraception and use abortion. More research is also needed on how cost affects the use of various contraceptives and abortion, allowing the development of strategies favoring contraception. Research to identify the consequences of induced abortion on subsequent reproductive function is necessary. Health system research on the impact and acceptability of new technologies of abortion might lead to better abortion services, reducing the morbidity related to abortion. However, regardless of the specific objective, research should be designed with policy change as the foremost goal (Rogow, 1989).

Recognizing the unique context and special needs of EE, the Special Programme of Research, Development and Research Training in Human Reproduction of the World Health Organization (HRP) established in 1994 a Scientific Working Group on Reproductive Health Research in Eastern Europe. With the collaboration of scientists from EE countries, the Group has identified priorities for research and training activities. The health consequences of abortion is one of the key elements of reproductive health that the research program is focusing on. Several multicenter research projects address different topics in this area in EE countries, like the determinants of choice and use of fertility regulation methods (Project 95905), morbidity after induced abortion (Project 95910), and the impact on service delivery of the introduction of a medical abortion technology (Project 95906). Another important objective of the Group is seeking to establish an East–West scientific collaboration between centers and scientists working in reproductive health. There are many well trained researchers in EE countries who have great potential for collaboration with their Western counterparts, and these resources may be extremely useful in identifying the needs, and in designing and conducting the research required to address the reproductive health problems in the subregion (UNDP/UNFPA/WHO/World Bank Special Programme of Research, Development and Research Training in Human Reproduction, 1995).

Conclusions

Chapter 8, Paragraph 25 of the ICPD Program of Action states that: "Prevention of unwanted pregnancies must always be given the highest priority and all attempts should be made to eliminate the need for abortion" (UN, 1995a). Based on the new approach promoted by this important conference, a broadening of the concept of reproductive health must be understood and applied in EE countries. Reproductive health means more than the mere absence of disease, and it must be restored, protected, and promoted not only by medical interventions, but also by economic, social, and educational interventions. Good reproductive health for all must be achieved through a comprehensive and integrated approach that places emphasis on people not problems. This approach should start with a documentation of the needs and perspectives of the different parties involved (women, teenagers, communities, medical providers, educators, policymakers) as a prerequisite to identifying problems and formulating new strategies to address them.

In an attempt to summarize an answer to the question in the title of this paper, "how can the rates of induced abortion be reduced?", it can be stated that prevention of unwanted pregnancies through information, education, and access to modern contraception is the most effective strategy for decreasing the rate of induced abortions. This strategy is also considered to be one of the most efficient and essential health interventions that can improve women's health, conferring widespread economic and social benefits (The World Bank, 1994). It was estimated that the economic effect of reducing the number of abortions in the Russian Federation by 15–20% would generate 165 million roubles annually (Komyssova, 1992).

Although it may be a long process (Hassoun, and Jourdain, 1995), EE countries must shift from "post-factum" to preventive family planning strategies, from an "abortion culture" to a "contraception culture." Abortion must not be promoted as an instrument of family planning and fertility regulation (The Szeged Declaration, 1994), but it should be recognized as an important component of reproductive health. Where national policies permit, it must be included in all programs that promote women's health, because the provision of good abortion services is an important factor in reducing abortion-related mortality and morbidity (Sundström, 1993; The World Bank, 1994).

It must be understood, however, that although the incidence of abortion in EE can be reduced over time, by combined national and international efforts, it cannot be eliminated altogether, given the shortcomings of current contraceptive methods, the possible human failings of users, and the inevitable fact that some women's life situations may change after the onset of a pregnancy. Therefore the issue of abortion must remain a priority for EE governments and international agencies.

Solutions to the abortion issue are only partially medical, they are mainly economic, social and educational. Such a conclusion is not surprising, given the complexity of this subject, which was comprehensively summarized almost 20 years ago by Christopher Tietze as follows: "Abortion is more than a medical issue, or an ethical issue, or a legal issue. It is, above all, a human issue, involving women and men as individuals, as couples, and as members of societies."

Acknowledgments

The author gratefully acknowledges the helpful advice of the following individuals who reviewed all or parts of this paper and offered their thoughtful comments on the manuscript: Brooke R. Johnson, Harrison McKay, Eva Mathur, and Constantin Enciulescu.

References

Atrash, H. K., and Hogue, C. J. R. 1990. The effect of pregnancy termination on future reproduction. *Bailliere's Clinical Obstetrics and Gynecology* 4:391–405.

Berbik, I. 1994. New Hungarian abortion act: first results. *Planned Parenthood in Europe* 23:24–5.

Benson Gold, R. 1990. *Abortion and women's health.* New York: Allen Guttmacher Institute.

Bostandjiev, R. 1992. Sexual education in transition in Bulgaria. *Planned Parenthood in Europe* 22:13–4.

Bruyniks, N. P. 1994. Reproductive health in Central and Eastern Europe: priorities and needs. *Patient Education and Counseling* 23:203–15.

Chudikova, A. 1992. Reproductive health challenges in the Slovak Republic. *Planned Parenthood in Europe* 22:27.

Cook, R. J. 1993. From abortion to reproductive health—the role of the law. In *Progress postponed: abortion in Europe in the 1990s.* 60–77. London: International Planned Parenthood Federation

Cottingham. J., and Mehta, S. 1993. Medical barriers to contraceptive use. *Reproductive Health Matters* 1:97–100.

Czech Statistical Office, Factum, non fabula, Institute for the Care of Mother and Child Prague and Center for Disease Control and Prevention Atlanta. 1995. *Czech Republic reproductive health survey 1993—final report.* Prague: Czech Statistical Office.

David, H. P. 1992. Abortion in Europe, 1920–91: a public health perspective. *Studies in Family Planning* 23:1–22.

David, H. P., and Baban, A. 1996. Women's health and reproductive rights: Romanian experience. *Patient Education and Counseling* 28:235–45.

Djusubalieva, T. 1994. Reproductive health in Kazakhstan: a new approach. *Planned Parenthood in Europe* 23:17–19.

Frejka, T. 1983. Induced abortion and fertility: a quarter century of experience in Eastern Europe. *Population and Development Review* 9:494–520.

Frejka, T. 1990. *Issues of reproductive health: contraception and induced abortion in Central and Eastern Europe.* Presentation at the Annual Meeting of the American Public Health Association.

Grebsheva, I. 1992. Abortion and the problem of family planning in Russia. *Planned Parenthood in Europe* 21:8–9.

Greenslade, F. C., Early McLaurin, K., Leonard, A., Winkler, J., and Bhiwandiwala, P. 1993. Technology introduction and quality of abortion care. *Journal of Women's Health* 2:27–33.

Hassoun, D., and Jourdain, A. 1995. Contraception et avortement dans les pays d'Europe de l'Est. *Cahiers de Sociologie et de Démographie Médicales* 35:99–123.

Henshaw, S., and Morrow, E. 1990. *Induced abortion. A world review 1990 supplement.* New York: Allen Guttmacher Institute.

Hogue, C. J. 1986. Impact of abortion on subsequent fecundity. *Clinical Obstetrics and Gynecology* 13:95–103.

Holmgren, K., and Uddenberg, N. 1994. Abortion ethics—women's post abortion assessments. *Acta Obstetricia et Gynecologica Scandinavica* 73:1–5.

Hord, C., and David, H. P., Donnay, F., and Wolf, M. 1991. Reproductive health in Romania: reversing the Ceausescu legacy. *Studies in Family Planning* 22:231–240.

121

IOMC and CDC. 1995. Reproductive health survey, Romania, 1993—final report. Bucharest: Institute for Mother and Child Care Bucharest and Centers for Disease Control and Prevention Atlanta.

IPPF. 1989. International Planned Parenthood Federation, Europe Region, and Mouvement Français pour le Planning Familial France. Late abortion in Europe. Facing the problem–Causes–Prevention. Report of a colloquium. London: International Planned Parenthood Federation, Europe Region.

Jacobson, J. L. 1990. The global politics of abortion. *Worldwatch Paper 97.* Washington, DC: Worldwatch Institute.

Johnson, B. R., Benson, J., Bradley, J., Rabago Ordoñez, A., Zambrano, C., Okoko, L., Vázquez Chávez, L., Quiroz, P., and Rogo, K. 1993a. Costs of alternative treatments for incomplete abortion. *The World Bank, Population and Human Resources Department, Policy research working paper WPS 1072.* Washington, DC: The World Bank.

Johnson, B. R., Horga, M., and Andronache, L. 1993b. Contraception and abortion in Romania. *Lancet* 341:875–78.

Johnson, B. R., Horga, M., and Andronache, L. 1996. Women's perspectives on abortion in Romania. *Social Science and Medicine* 42:521–530.

Ketting, E., Lehert, P., Uzel, R., and Visser, A. 1992. Contraceptive practices and attitudes of women in the Czech and Slovak Federal Republic. *Planned Parenthood in Europe* 22:14–18.

Khomassuridze, A. 1994. Family planning in Georgia: a continued struggle. *Planned Parenthood in Europe* 23:17–9.

Kligman, G. 1992. The politics of reproduction in Ceausescu's Romania: a case study in political culture. *East European Politics and Societies* 6:364–418.

Komyssova, N. 1992. Family planning in the Russian Federation. *Planned Parenthood in Europe* 21:7–8.

Koontz, S. L., and Conly, S.R. 1993. *Expanding access to safe abortion: key policy issues,* 8. Washington DC: Population Action International Information Kit.

Leonard, A. H., and Ladipo, O. A. 1994. Post-abortion family planning: factors in individual choice of contraceptive methods. *IPAS Advances in Abortion Care*, 4:1–4.

Liskin, L. S. 1980. Complications of abortion in developing countries. *Population Reports* Series F, No. 7.

Nowicka, W. 1993a. The new abortion law in Poland. *Planned Parenthood in Europe* 22:21–24.

Nowicka, W. 1993b. Two steps back: Poland's new abortion law. *Planned Parenthood in Europe* 22:18–20.

122

Popov, A. A. 1993. A short history of abortion and population policy in Russia. *Planned Parenthood in Europe* 22:23–25.

Popov, A. A, Visser, A. P, and Ketting, E. 1993. Contraceptive knowledge, attitudes, and practice in Russia during the 1980s. *Studies in Family Planning* 24:227–235.

Rogow, D. 1989. Designing abortion research for policy impact. In *Methodological issues in abortion research. Proceedings of a seminar presented under the Population Council's Robert H. Ebert Program on Critical Issues in Reproductive Health.* 110–114. New York: The Population Council,

Sahatci, E. 1993a. Abortion and women's health in Albania. *Planned Parenthood in Europe* 22:20–1.

Sahatci, E. 1993b. Albania discovers the human right to family planning. *Planned Parenthood in Europe* 22:25–6.

Segal, S. J., and LaGuardia, K. D. 1990. Termination of pregnancy—a global view. *Bailliere's Clinical Obstetrics and Gynaecology*, 4:235–47.

Serbanescu, F., Morris, L., Stupp, P., and Stanescu, A. 1995. The impact of recent policy changes on fertility, abortion, and contraceptive use in Romania. *Planned Parenthood in Europe* 26:76–87.

Shah, I. 1996. *Fertility and contraception in Europe.* Presentation at the Fourth Meeting of the Scientific Working Group on Reproductive Health Research in Eastern Europe, Tirgu Mures, Romania.

Spinelli, A., Figa-Talamanca, I., and David, H. 1993. Psychosocial effects of early and late induced abortions. In *Progress postponed: abortion in Europe in the 1990,* 126–147. London: International Planned Parenthood Federation, Europe Region.

Stephenson, P., Wagner, M., Badea, M., and Serbanescu, F. 1992. Commentary: the public health consequences of restricted induced abortion—lessons from Romania. *American Journal of Public Health*, 82:1328–31.

Sundström, K. 1993. Abortion: a reproductive health issue. Working paper prepared for the World Bank's Women's Health and Nutrition Work Program.

Tbilisi Declaration. 1990. Issued by the international conference "From abortion to contraception", Tbilisi, 1990.

The Allen Guttmacher Institute. 1995. *Hopes and realities. Closing the gap between women's aspirations and their reproductive experiences.* New York: The Allen Guttmacher Institute.

The Szeged Declaration. 1994. Assessment of research and service needs on reproductive health in Eastern Europe—concern and commitments. *Human Reproduction,* 9: 750–752.

The World Bank. 1994. *Development in practice. A new agenda for women's health and nutrition*. Washington, DC: The World Bank.

UN, Department for Economic and Social Information and Policy Analysis, Population Division. 1994. *World contraceptive use 1994*. New York: United Nations.

UN. 1995a. *The Programme of Action of the International Conference on Population and Development, Cairo, 1994*. New York: United Nations.

UN, Department for Economic and Social Information and Policy Analysis, Population Division. 1995b. *World population prospects, The 1994 revision*. 135. New York: United Nations.

UNDP/UNFPA/WHO/World Bank Special Programme of Research, Development and Research Training in Human Reproduction. 1994. *Biennial report 1992–1993*. Geneva: World Health Organization.

UNDP/UNFPA/WHO/World Bank Special Programme of Research, Development and Research Training in Human Reproduction. 1995. *Annual technical report 1995*. Geneva: World Health Organization.

UNFPA. 1995. *Report of the Workshop on the implementation of the Cairo Programme of Action in countries with economies in transition, Sinaia, Romania, 1995*. United Nations Population Fund.

Visser, A. P., Pavlenko, I., Remmenick, L., Bruyniks, N., and Lehert, P. 1993a. Contraceptive practice and attitudes in former Soviet women. *Advances in Contraception* 9:13–23.

Visser, A. P., Bruyniks, N., and Remmenick, L. 1993b. Family planning in Russia: experience and attitude of gynecologists. *Advances in Contraception* 9:93–104.

Visser, A. P., Remenninck, L., and Bruyniks, N. 1993c. Contraception in Russia: attitude, knowledge and practice of doctors. *Planned Parenthood in Europe* 1993, 22:26–29.

Visser, A., Uzel, R., Ketting, E., Bruyniks, N., and Oddens, B. 1994. Practice, attitudes and knowledge of Czech and Slovak gynecologists concerning contraception. *Planned Parenthood in Europe* 23:19–23.

Wolf, M. 1994. Consequences and prevention of induced abortion. *IPAS Issues in Abortion Care* 3:5–17.

Wolf, M., and Benson, J. 1994. Meeting women's needs for post-abortion family planning. Report of a Bellagio Technical Working Group. *International Journal of Gynaecology and Obstetrics* 45 (Suppl.): 3–23.

WHO. 1993. *World health statistics yearbook*. Geneva: World Health Organization.

WHO. 1994. *WHO Scientific Group on Medical Methods for Termination of Pregnancy*. Medical methods for termination of pregnancy: report of a WHO

124

scientific group. Geneva: World Health Organization. (WHO Technical Report Series, No. 871.)

WHO. 1995a. *Complications of abortion. Technical and managerial guidelines for prevention and treatment.* Geneva: World Health Organization.

WHO. 1995b. *The world health report 1995.* Geneva: World Health Organization.

WHO Regional Office for Europe and United Nations Population Fund. 1995. *From abortion to contraception. Family planning and reproductive health in CCEE/NIS.* Copenhagen: World Health Organization.

Table 6.1

Fertility, birth, abortion, and contraception prevalence rates in countries
of Eastern Europe

Source: WHO and United Nations Population Fund (1995)

Country	Total fertility rate (/woman)	Birthrate (/1000 population)	Abortion rate (/1000 women of fertile age)	Abortion to birth ratio	Contraceptive prevalence rate (/100 women of fertile age)
Albania	3^e	23^e	17^c	0.35^b	10^e
Armenia	2.6^e	21^e	29.6^b	0.36^c	10^b
Azerbaijan	2.7^e	26^e	239^d	2.3^d	7^e
Belarus	1.7^e	12^e	85.9^c	1.64^c	30^c
Bosnia and Herzegovina	1.6^e	14^e	112^d	2^d	
Bulgaria	1.5^e	10.5^d		1.44^b	22^c
Croatia	1.4^e	10^e	27.2^d	0.65^d	
Czech Republic	1.7^e	12^e	41.5^c	0.77^c	38^e
Estonia	1.5^e	10^e	66.3^e	1.49^e	26^c
Federal Republic of Yugoslavia	1.9^e	14^e			
Former Yugoslav Republic of Macedonia	1.9^e	16^e	54.4^e	0.85^e	39^e
Georgia	2.2^e	17^e	41.1^c	0.59^c	19^c
Hungary	1.7^e	11^e	33.3^c	0.76^d	62^c
Kazakhstan	2.8^e	20^e	70.4^e	0.88^e	22^e
Kyrgyzstan	3.7^e	26.9^d	58.8^e	0.5^e	25^e
Latvia	1.7^e	12^e	70.4^a	1.29^e	19^d
Lithuania	1.9^e	14^e	29.7^a	0.51^c	12^c
Moldova	2.1^e	13^e	74.6^d	1.43^d	24^d
Poland	2.1^d	14.5^d	14^c	0.22^c	26^c
Romania	1.4^e	11.4^c	138.4^c	2.7^c	11^d
Russia	1.6^e	11^e	98.1^c	2.24^c	22^c
Slovakia	1.9^e	14^e	31.6^d	0.7^d	38^c
Slovenia	1.3^e	10^e	28^c	0.7^d	40^d
Tajikistan	5^e	33^d	39.6^d	0.3^d	15^e
Turkmenistan	4.1^e	33.1^e	31.4^e	0.24^e	19^e
Ukraine	1.7^e	12^e	82^a	1.5^a	17^a
Uzbekistan	4.4^e	33^e			19^e

[a]1990, [b]1991, [c]1992, [d]1993, [e]1994

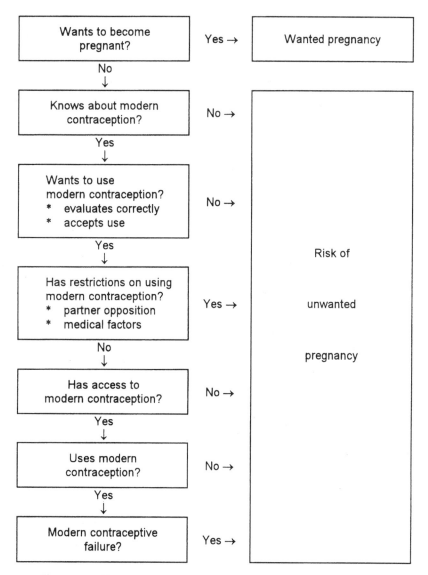

Figure 6.1. Flowchart of the process resulting in a woman having an unwanted pregnancy.

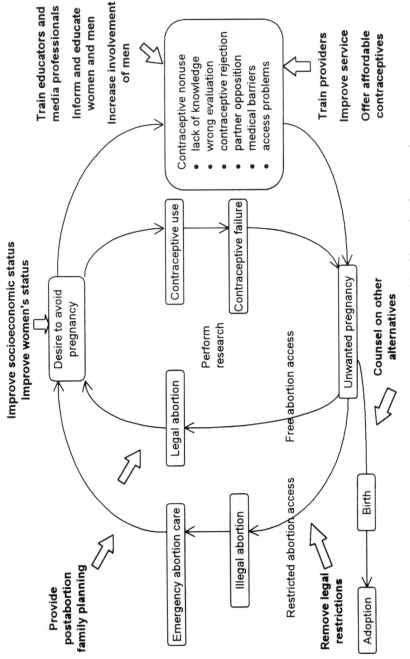

Figure 6.2. Strategies to reduce abortion rates by breaking the cycle of unwanted pregnancy.

128

Infertility in Eastern Europe: a survey of the current status in nine countries

FRANK LÜDICKE,[1] ASSIA BRANDRUP-LUKANOW,[2]
MIHAI HORGA[3] and ALDO CAMPANA[1]

[1] WHO Collaborating Center for Research in Human Reproduction, Clinic for Infertility and Gynaecological Endocrinology, University Hospital, Geneva, Switzerland;
[2] WHO Regional Office for Europe, Sexual and Family Health Unit, Copenhagen, Denmark; [3] Center of Public Health, Targu-Mures, Romania

Abstract

A questionnaire survey was conducted among clinics of obstetrics and gynecology in the countries of Eastern Europe and the Newly Independent States that attempted to assess information on the medical infrastructure for infertility, sources of information, type of equipment and facilities in place, investigations performed, and the evaluation of the characteristics of the infertile couple. Information on nine countries in the region was collected, which revealed that in each country at least one referral center for infertility existed and that all centers were in principle equipped to perform the necessary investigations. A large number of cases of tubal damage was reported and a considerable number of pregnancy and postabortion complications. It is hypothesized that postabortion infections contribute significantly to infertility problems in the region. There was a large disparity between detected female/male causes, which is most likely due to the fact that a standardized approach for the male was not yet established in these services.

Introduction

The reasons for infertility are different in different regions in the world and infertility is particularly high in countries with a high incidence of sexually transmitted diseases (STDs) (WHO, 1975). It is believed that the rate of infertility in countries in Eastern Europe and in the Newly Independent States (EE/NIS) is in the same range as in countries of Western Europe—namely, 10% (WHO, 1991). In fact, the data on infertility in the region are sparse and consistent epidemiological evidence is lacking.

The political, economic, and sociocultural revolution in these countries has resulted in a period of social instability, and the desire for birth control became a primary aim to many individuals. The fertility rate fell below the replacement level in a number of societies in EE/NIS, and this is often produced by induced abortion. When we talk to medical health professionals in the region, it seems that there is a consensus that the high rate of abortion is largely responsible for secondary infertility. Induced abortions, performed in suboptimal settings, because of high caseloads and a lack of medical sustainables (like e.g. diagnostic kits), could lead to postabortion complications and, therefore, contribute to subsequent infertility. Thus, the question of multiple abortions (which is common in EE/NIS) and subsequent infertility has not been adequately addressed until now and requires more work. Maternal mortality is still high in countries like Russia and Albania (about 50 per 100 000 livebirths) and mainly attributable to the complications of abortion (WHO and UN Population Fund, 1995). Moreover, some articles report high postabortion infection rates (Bruyniks, 1994). This reinforces the hypothesis of infertility linked to abortion as it is practiced in EE/NIS.

With the rise in the incidence of STDs in the region (see also the paper by Dr. Gromyko in this publication) and the apparent toxic environmental effects on reproduction in certain areas of

EE/NIS (Kulin, and Skakkebaek, 1995), there are two other risk factors that may negatively affect fertility.

In view of the fact that many women, confronted with precarious social conditions, postpone having their first child to later years, it became even more important than in the past to have the possibility of deciding when to give birth to a child. Thus, access to effective contraceptive methods and the avoidance and treatment of unwanted infertility constitute basic reproductive rights, which are of increasing importance to the region and all efforts should be made to empower these women.

As a first approach to a better understanding of infertility in EE/NIS, a survey was conducted in a number of selected centers. It was hoped that the information gathered would provide a clearer picture, at least for some countries, of this still poorly investigated area of reproductive health in EE/NIS and that it could trigger future collaborative programs.

Materials and methods

A questionnaire survey was conducted among the heads of departments of obstetrics and gynecology (mostly WHO Collaborating Centers) in 15 countries of EE/NIS. The questionnaires were designed to obtain information on the medical infrastructure within the country for infertility, on sources of recent medical information, on type of equipment and facilities in place, on investigations performed, and on the characteristics of infertile couples. The information that was asked for was from the completed year 1995. The percentages given for the total results are calculated as an average from percentages from each center. The heads of departments or an appropriate member of staff were asked to complete the questionnaire in English. Contributors from each country are listed at the end of the article. The questionnaires were sent out in November 1996.

Results

Eighteen out of the 30 centers to which the questionnaire was sent responded. All centers were teaching hospitals with the exception of one. Information from nine different countries was collected. In each of the countries listed at least one specialized service for infertility existed (table 7.1). Several centers reported an extraordinarily high number of cases of infertility (table 7.1). It should be noted that clinics in Georgia and Moldavia, for example, are the only national referral centers in their countries. Professional associations dealing with infertility are reported to be in Hungary, the Russian Federation, and recently in Romania. Specific national legislation or recommendations as regards donor insemination and adoption of children existed in seven of the countries.

The main sources of information on reproductive health were reported to be WHO publications, scientific journals, and travel to international congresses. The Internet was used by a minority of centers. Access to the Internet was reported in two of the nine countries only.

The Task Force on the Prevention and Management of Infertility, Special Programme of Research in Human Reproduction (HRP/ WHO) has developed a standardized approach to the investigation of infertile couples (Rowe et al., 1993). According to this approach, the following investigations are required in women: general and gynecological examination, detection of ovulation, and laparoscopy, and optional investigations are in hysterosalpingography, hormonal status, and the postcoital test. In the male partner a general physical and andrological examination and semen analysis were defined as a minimal requirement, whereas hormonal status was considered to be supplementary.

A general physical examination and gynecological examination are standard in all centers and an andrological examination and semen analysis were routinely carried out in all men investigated.

Detection of ovulation was standard in all centers. The majority used a basal body temperature chart and ultrasound. Measurements of progesterone concentrations were made in 66% of the centers.

Hysterosalpingography is the preferred method for the routine infertility work-up in comparison with laparoscopy with the tubal patency test. In 22% of the centers neither method is done routinely. The postcoital test was carried out routinely in all of the clinics (table 7.2). Of the clinics that performed semen analysis, all adhered to the WHO recommendation on normal sperm count —namely, $\geq 20 \times 10^6$ spermatozoa/ml and a motility $\geq 50\%$.

All the centers had antibiotics for the treatment of genital tract infections, including STDs, at their disposal, but only in 50% of centers was a routine test used for *Chlamydia* infection. In all centers ovarian stimulation was performed in indicated cases. Donor insemination can be performed in the countries concerned. Intrauterine insemination with the husband's sperm is practiced in cases of a diagnosis of a male or cervical factor. In vitro fertilization was available in all countries with the exception of Armenia and Uzbekistan (table 7.3).

Overall, the characteristics of the couples and the distribution patterns of the causes of infertility were recorded in 79 600 cases. The majority of women who consulted for infertility were aged 25 to 34 years and more often they presented primary infertility. The duration of time before a couple seeks medical aid in EE/NIS was longer compared to countries with fully developed economies. While in Western countries 45% of couples wait less than two years before consulting the medical services (Cates, 1988), only 15% of couples do so in EE/NIS (table 7.4). A large number of pregnancy and postabortion complications, infections, and traumatic complications were reported. In their medical history 35% of the women had had one of these conditions; 35% of women (table 7.5) and 42% of men had a previous history of an STD.

133

Concerning the causes of infertility, these were detected twice as often in women than in men. Causes found in both were attributed to 25% of cases. Unexplained infertility was present in 10% of cases (table 7.6). Table 7.7 gives the pattern of causes of infertility as reported by the centers. Bilateral or unilateral tubal occlusion and pelvic adhesions make up more than half of the female causes. Infection-related causes in men were found in 18%. The likelihood of detecting a cause in women was much higher than in men. In 12% of the women, no specific diagnosis was established, and this was the case in 45% of the men.

Discussion

It is understood that this survey can only give a crude view of the issue and is by no means representative of the whole region or even of a single country. The main restriction was the limited number of centers included in the survey and the fact that we had no control on how the different centers reached a diagnosis of infertility. Despite these limitations, some hypotheses and trends can be drawn from the results.

In all the countries of EE/NIS represented in this survey specialized services existed for infertility. Unlike in Western European countries, only a few governments have issued special laws or guidelines concerning infertility treatment. Donor insemination is available, and adoption as an option to overcome childlessness is regulated by law in all countries.

Most of the participating centers were reasonably well equipped. Ultrasonography, hysterosalpingography, and semen analysis were available. Hormonal status could be determined in indicated cases. Laparoscopy was available in 80% of the centers, but, contrary to the WHO recommendations and as in many centers in Western Europe (Helmerhorst et al., 1995), was not routinely performed. Endometriosis can only be diagnosed by direct inspection of the pelvic organs, therefore, we have good reason to believe that endometriosis as a cause of infertility is underestimated in our figures.

There was a large disparity in reported female/male causes, which is most likely due to the fact that men have not yet sufficiently entered into the picture of the management of infertility in these services and a standardized approach for the male was not yet established. This may be a cultural matter, but it was noted, too, that the discipline of andrology warrants more development in EE/NIS in future (Kulin, and Skakkebaek, 1995).

Genital infection seems to have an important role in EE/NIS. The frequency of infection-related diagnoses in the female (tubal damage and pelvic adhesions) would place EE/NIS in relation to other regions in the world second behind Africa and before Asia, Latin America, and the developed world (Cates et al., 1988). A considerable number of women also reported postabortion complications. It is plausible that postabortion infections contribute significantly to infertility in the region. Moreover, it can be assumed that in most countries of EE/NIS, where the anticipated family size of one or two children is reached at a young age, the inherent risk of repeated abortions on fertility will not be obvious.

Treatment of infection was available in all centers. Intrauterine insemination and ovarian stimulation was done in indicated cases. Treatment possibilities for bilateral tubal occlusion were found to be limited. Microsurgery and in vitro fertilization are just beginning to be performed in EE/NIS.

Worldwide, some form of infertility affects at least 8 to 12% of couples during their reproductive life, which is about 50 to 80 million people. In any single population sterility affects at least 3 to 5% of couples.

From a public health point of view, the best use of limited financial resources to defeat infertility and sterility is the prevention of STDs. Many governments, international agencies and non governmental organizations have, therefore, prioritized preven-

135

tive programs for their activities and allocation of funds. The United Nations Fund for Population Activities (UNFPA) has defined its assistance in this field to activities like simple diagnostic screening to identify the cause of infertility, treatment for STDs associated with infertility, education, and counseling aimed to prevent STDs, and related training activities (Sabwa, 1994).

Equally important for preventing infertility are the practice of safe procedures in places where induced abortions are performed and good services for the management of complications arising from abortion (ICPD, 1994). Safe abortion, performed under proper conditions, reduces the frequency of pelvic inflammatory disease (PID) and cervical and uterine damage, which are established risk factors for subsequent infertility.

The use of contraceptive methods per se is a preventive measure for infertility. Hormonal methods reduce the risk of PID. Barrier methods, in particular condom use, provide protection against STDs. In general, all contraceptive methods lessen the frequency of unwanted pregnancies and, therefore, the number of abortions.

As in any other case, prevention is better than cure. Often, however, the subject of the treatment of infertility is dealt with in a negative manner. There is a plethora of articles informing the reader about how costly the investigation and treatment of infertility is, and how depressing its success rates can be. Some tend to adopt a slightly abstract point of view in declaring that the number of children born as the result of the treatment of infertility is marginal in relation to the problem of overpopulation (Vekemans, 1994).

Rational policy and constraints in the national health budgets in countries of economies in transition like in EE/NIS make it meaningful to integrate STD prevention programs into primary health care and family planning services rather than to establish specialized infertility services. However, in many of these countries, the medical infrastructure is well developed with well-trained professionals. Methods like laparoscopy, which were regarded as a luxury just a few years ago, are spreading rapidly and are also used in low-budget environments. The development of nonisotopic hormone assays make the laboratory equipment less demanding and the existing guidelines on the minimal and rational management of the infertile couple render the infertility work-up more effective (WHO, 1980; Rowe et al., 1993). From the health perspective, which is not merely the absence of disease or infirmity, but also the mental, social, and physical well-being of the individual, and that of the magnitude of the problem, infertility treatment claims a legitimate place in publicly financed health services. This should be based on the principle of equitable distribution of resources according to the magnitude of a problem, the feasibility of successful treatment, and the scientific and moral obligation to expand access to modern technology and the benefits of scientific innovation to those who need it (Shah, 1994).

The diagnosis and treatment of infertility take a secondary role in comparison to preventing infertility, but there is merit in giving some thought to building up or sustaining a few centers of excellence in the region that can address the sensitive issues of infertility and sterility.

This report of selected institutions in EE/NIS is only one small step in addressing the problem of infertility, which is of importance to many individuals in EE/NISO. For future collaborative efforts, we want to highlight the following areas of research and activity that address the problem of infertility in EE/NIS:

1. To obtain more precise and representative data on causes of infertility in the region and, in doing so, apply a standardized approach of management of the infertile couple. This will improve professional capacity within the centers and allow them to focus more on the male factor than might have been done in the past.

2. To assess the impact of environmental factors that affect fertility in the region and to inform policymakers about the results.

3. To assess and perform research on the impact of multiple abortions, on the current practices of abortion services, as well as the incidence of pregnancy complications, and to act by improving service delivery and thereby reduce puerperal and postabortion infections.

4. To evaluate the impact of STD prevention programs aiming at defining appropriate STD prevention strategies in the region and to advocate the implementation of such STD prevention programs.

5. To assess the factors which result in low use of modern contraception and to take action by strengthening family planning programs and to overcome obstacles that hamper contraceptive use and, therefore, may lead to unwanted pregnancy and abortion.

Acknowledgments

We are grateful to Dr. Tomas Frejka, United Nations Economic Commission for Europe; Dr. Helena Honkanen, WHO Special Programme of Research, Development and Research Training in Human Reproduction; Dr. Gunilla Lindmark, WHO Collaborating Center for Research in Human Reproduction Uppsala; and Eva Mathur, WHO Collaborating Center for Research in Human Reproduction Geneva, for their contributions to the document, and to our colleagues in Eastern Europe and the Newly Independent States who kindly completed and returned the questionnaires.

References

Bruyniks, N. P. 1994. Reproductive health in Central and Eastern Europe: priorities and needs. *Patient Education and Counseling* 23:203–15.

Cates, W., Farley, T. M. M., and Rowe, P. J. 1988. Patterns of infertility in the developed and developing worlds. In *Diagnosis and treatment of infertility,* eds. P. J. Rowe, and E. M. Vikhlyaeva, 57. Bern: Hans Huber.

Helmerhorst, F. M., Oei, S. G., Bloemenkamp, K. W. M., and Keirse, M. J. N. C. 1995. Consistency and variation infertility investigations in Europe. *Human Reproduction* 8: 2027–30.

Kulin, H. E., and Skakkebaek, N. E. 1995. Environmental effects on human reproduction: the basis for new efforts in Eastern Europe. *Social Science and Medicine* 41: 1479–86.

Rowe, P. J., Comhaire, F. H., Hargreave, T. B., and Mellows, H. J. 1993. *WHO manual for the standardized investigation and diagnosis of the infertile couple.* Cambridge: Cambridge University Press.

Sabwa, M. 1994. The role of UNFPA's involvement in the management of infertility: prevention and treatment. *Entre Nous, The European Family Planning Magazine;* 25

Shah, I. 1994. Treatment of infertility: an integral part of reproductive health and a necessity. *Reproductive Health Matters* 4: 96–97

UN. 1995. *The Program of Action of the International Conference on Population and Development, Cairo, 1994,* paragraph 8.25. New York: United Nations.

Vekemans, M. 1994. Is the treatment of infertility a luxury in a world in the middle of a population expansion? *Entre Nous, The European Family Planning Magazine;* 25:5.

WHO 1975. Scientific Group on the Epidemiology of Infertility. *The epidemiology of infertility.* Technical Report Series No. 582. Geneva: World Health Organization.

WHO 1980. Special Programme of Research, Development and Research Training in Human Reproduction. *Laboratory manual for the examination of human semen and semen cervical mucus interaction.* Singapore: Press Concern.

WHO 1991. *Infertility: a tabulation of available data on prevalence of primary and secondary infertility.* WHO/MCH 91.9. Geneva: World Health Organization.

WHO Regional Office for Europe and United Nations Population Fund. 1995. *Family planning and reproductive health in CCEE/NIS.* Copenhagen: World Health Organization.

Table 7.1

Existence of referral centers and national organizations dealing with infertility;
specific legislation on donor insemination or adoption in selected countries of EE/NIS

Country (No. of centers; no. of cases)	Existence of referral centers	National organization	Legislation on donor insemination	Legislation on adoption
Armenia (1; 70)	Yes	No	No	Yes
Bulgaria (1; 3500)	Yes	No	Yes	Yes
Georgia (1; 8372)	Yes	No	Yes	Yes
Hungary (2; 11 970)	Yes	Yes	Yes	Yes
Kazakhstan (1; 7973)	Yes	No	Yes	Yes
Republic of Moldova (1; 35 000)	Yes	No	No	Yes
Romania (9; 7503)	Yes	Yes	No	Yes
Russian Federation (1; 4300)	Yes	Yes	No	Yes
Uzbekistan (1; 912)	Yes	No	No	Yes

Table 7.2

Investigation of infertility as performed by the centers in nine countries of EE/NIS (%)

	Routinely	When indicated	Not provided
In the male			
General physical examination	100		
Andrological examination	100		
Semen analysis	100		
Hormonal status		100	
In the female			
General physical examination	100		
Gynecological examination	100		
Ovulation detection	100		
Laparoscopy + dye	12	66	22
Hormonal status		100	
Postcoital test	100		
Hysterosalpingography	77	33	
In vitro			
Sperm-cervical mucus contact test		100	

Table 7.3

Possible treatments offered by the centers in nine countries of EE/NIS (%)

Antibiotics for treatment of infections	100
Bromocriptine	100
Ovarian stimulation	100
Intrauterine insemination	100
Donor insemination	88
Laparoscopic surgery	65
Microsurgery	86
In vitro fertilization	77

Table 7.4

Age distribution and type of infertility (%)

(N= 79 600)

Age of woman (years)	
≤ 24	14
25–34	75
> 35	11
Age of man (years)	
≤ 24	4
25–34	62
> 35	34
Type of infertility	
Female primary	65
Female secondary	35
Male primary	70
Male secondary	30
Duration of infertility (years)	
≤ 2	15
2–4	70
> 4	15

Table 7.5

Self-reported history, female partner (%) (N= 79 600)

Previous history of sexually transmitted disease	35
Pregnancy complications	11
Postabortion complications	24

141

Table 7.6

General categories of infertility (%)

No cause found in either	10
Female cause only	44
Male cause only	21
Causes found in both	25

Table 7.7

Distribution of specific diagnoses of infertility (% diagnoses)

Female diagnosis

No demonstrable cause	12
Bilateral tubal occlusion	24
Unilateral tubal occlusion	10
Pelvic adhesions	17
Ovulatory failure	18
Hyperprolactinemia	3
Endometriosis	3
Acquired uterine or cervical lesions	5
Missing data	8

Male diagnosis

No demonstrable cause	45
Varicocele	5
Accessory gland infection	18
Idiopathic oligo-, astheno-, terato-, or azoospermia	8
Missing data	24

142

Towards better reproductive health in Eastern Europe

ASSIA BRANDRUP-LUKANOW

WHO Regional Office for Europe, Sexual and Family Health Unit,
Copenhagen, Denmark

Abstract

The period of transition in Eastern Europe and the Newly Independent States particularly affected the health of women and children. Strategies for change to improve this situation include training of health professionals and a multidisciplinary approach. Data show high rates of maternal and infant mortality, high ratios of abortions to livebirths, and low use of modern methods of family planning with a preference for intrauterine devices, while barrier methods are hardly used at all. In view of the increasing epidemic of AIDS and sexually transmitted diseases, and the lack of knowledge about reproductive health among the population and particularly among teenagers, it is important that strategies of cooperation are developed between the health sector and the education and information sectors. Data also show rising mortality from cancer of the cervix and from breast cancer. Screening programs should be incorporated into reproductive health and primary health care services.

Introduction

We have looked at the status of reproductive health in the Eastern region of Europe. It is clear that the indicators are much worse than in Western Europe. This applies to straightforward indicators of

143

mortality: maternal mortality is 2 to 12 times as high as in Western Europe, on average 7 times as high. Infant mortality, an indicator reflecting the quality of neonatal and obstetric care as well as the health of the mother prior to and during pregnancy and the quality of antenatal care, is up to 20 times higher than in Western Europe. Among the causes of maternal mortality, obstetric hemorrhage, sepsis, and toxicosis are highest.

Socioeconomic factors contribute significantly to the poor state of maternal and child health in the region. Ministries of health have very low budgets for public health expenditure, and in many countries health professionals are working for long periods of time without receiving any salary at all. High rates of maternal mortality are related to a lack of essential drugs at the primary health care level, a lack of updated obstetric equipment, a lack of transport facilities for the transport of high risk cases, and to problems related to outdated medical practices and skills among medical personnel.

Among the causes of infant mortality, acute respiratory and gastrointestinal diseases as well as perinatal complications rate relatively high. The concept of real interdisciplinary work between the obstetrician, the neonatologist, and the midwife during the perinatal period is still in its initial stages, and the practice of early breastfeeding and rooming-in (i.e. mother and baby being together in one hospital room) have only recently been introduced. Where they have been introduced, however, there are trends toward a decrease in postnatal complications in mothers (postpartum hemorrhage) and neonates (in particular acute respiratory infections).

In general, medical training, and particularly medical specialization, in Central and Eastern Europe and the Newly Independent States are relatively short compared to other European countries, and medical specialists have had little or no chance to update their knowledge through international exchanges. Though medical care covers all levels from the primary, paramedically staffed health post, to the tertiary level maternity hospital, referral practices were often such that high-risk cases would be kept a relatively long time at intermediate level centers before being transferred to adequately equipped hospitals, by which time it was often too late to help the patient. Antenatal care, for example, was extensive as far as the number of visits and physical examinations were concerned, but the limited diagnostic facilities available to the midwife often prevent timely recognition of a high-risk situation and timely referral.

Also, surveys of the existing health systems in Central and Eastern Europe show that there was an imbalance between the equipment of high-level republican (i.e. national level) centers, which often had very specialized laboratories and centers of intermediate or primary level, where even basic equipment could be lacking. In general, therefore, citizens of the capital and regional centers had access to better quality health care than citizens living in smaller towns and rural areas. This also explains the differences in mortality found between different regions within one country.

Of course, the mortality is only the tip of the iceberg. Other "softer" indicators than mortality are more difficult to measure. The extremely high abortion rates, as high as three abortions to one birth, the inverse of the Western European ratio (0.3:1) have consequences on women's morbidity. These range from the physical side effects of repeated surgical abortions to the elevated risk of infection and pelvic inflammatory disease, which may have a negative effect on subsequent fertility. In many countries of the Newly Independent States, though abortions are legal and performed under clinical conditions, deaths from abortion still explain about 15 to 20% of maternal mortality. This indicates that either abortions are on average performed late in the first trimester, so that complications are more frequent, or that the techniques are not state of the art, or that the drugs and equipment needed to treat complications are lacking. In many countries, vacuum aspirators are still lacking in small centers, and abortions are performed mainly by dilatation and curettage with old instruments which can no longer be properly sterilized.

Another cause of concern are the rising rates of teenage pregnancies and abortions. In Latvia, for example, induced abortions

145

in the under-19-year olds account for 10% of all registered abortions performed.

Where abortions are still the main method of regulating fertility, as in most countries of the region, the prevalence of modern contraceptives is low—as low as 5% in some of the Central Asian Republics, and only marginally higher in other regions of the Newly Independent States. Only Hungary and Slovakia have contraceptive prevalence rates that are comparable to those of Western Europe.

While controlling fertility by contraception or abortion remains the concern of a large majority of women of reproductive age, approximately 10% of couples seek medical help to solve problems of infertility. Overall, the percentage of infertile couples is comparable to that in other European countries; however, the etiology of infertility seems to differ. Postabortion complications may account for about 17% of causes of infertility, and ecological/toxic causes have an effect on male infertility.

The types of contraceptives used are limited, and among those used, intrauterine devices (IUDs) are used most, whereas barrier contraceptives such as male and female condoms, and chemical barriers, which could help in the prevention of sexually transmitted diseases as well as unwanted pregnancy, are hardly used at all.

This is partly due to the limited availability of contraceptives, due to their extremely high price. Where the average monthly salary is between $20 and $40, women cannot afford to pay between $2 and $5 for one cycle of oral contraceptives. Also, the continued supply of a certain type of contraceptive is not guaranteed. These factors may explain why many women prefer to use an IUD rather than other methods. The use of condoms is still limited, though there seems to be less resistance to them among men in Central and Eastern Europe than among men in Central Asia.

The limited use of barrier contraceptives is particularly worrying in view of the rising incidence of sexually transmitted diseases, especially syphilis and gonorrhea, and the expected rise in HIV infection. The examples from Latvia show that the incidence of syphilis among 15 to 17 year olds rose by 50% between 1994 and 1995. The dire economic circumstances and rising unemployment rates have forced many women into prostitution as a means of earning a family income. Though there are no official numbers, observations from various countries indicate that the proportion of adolescents among prostitutes is increasing.

The rising incidence of cervical cancer, in which sexually transmitted diseases are an important etiological factor, is beginning to become a matter of public health concern.

Screening programs for cervical cancer have been introduced in only a few of these countries, and some countries do not even have recourse to laboratories in which cytopathological diagnosis can be performed. In comparison, breast cancer rates are, so far, lower than in Western Europe; however, many countries are seeing rising breast cancer rates, paralleling the developments in Western Europe. Here, too, screening programs are still very limited and only a few countries have mammographic facilities available.

Strategies for change

In view of the dimensions of reproductive health problems in Central and Eastern Europe and the Newly Independent States, only a multifaceted and interdisciplinary strategy can lead to desired improvements and the realization of the "Health for All" targets set for the European Region.

The first step is to convince health policymakers that the investment in reproductive health will carry tangible public health rewards, and will result in a decrease of maternal and infant mortality and morbidity. The investment needed to be put into preventive reproductive health measures is far lower than that required for highly equipped centers of medically assisted pregnancy, which many countries are investing in at present.

147

Recent studies among women taking recourse to abortions in Russia have shown that the majority of them had not been informed on the use and availability of modern contraceptives. Information badly needs to be provided to not only the health service sector, but also to the media and the education sector. School health education curricula should be revised to include reproductive health. Information activities should also focus on promoting the use of condoms and other barrier methods.

Information should also particularly target high-risk groups, such as women seeking abortions. Postabortion counseling is badly needed and is still rarely found on a regular basis, due to the fact that the clinics are very busy and that medical professionals themselves are not trained in how to provide counseling.

Teenagers need a different type of information from adults. Age at first sexual intercourse is decreasing continuously and unwanted pregnancies in this young age group are most often the result of a first unprotected sexual contact. Information and counseling centers for adolescents should exist at least in the cities, but also in smaller towns in the rural areas, allowing young people to receive information anonymously and confidentiality.

Information activities targeting men need to be reinforced, particularly in view of the rise in sexually transmitted diseases and AIDS. Health education authorities should work closely with the media to maintain a high level of activity.

Regarding legal issues, examples from countries of Eastern Europe show that restricting abortions leads to a rise in illegally performed abortions and in maternal mortality, whereas the liberalization of abortion laws has led to a decrease in maternal mortality.

These are suggestions for strategies for family planning. This, however, is only one factor contributing to the reproductive health of women in Central and Eastern Europe. In order to combat the high rates of maternal mortality and morbidity, further efforts targeting the primary health care and obstetric services need to be made. Upgrading the skills of health professionals, bringing them in line with international standards, is the first requirement. In upgrading skills, it is important not only to target specialists working in referral hospitals, but also particularly those medical workers who provide primary health care, be they general practitioners or midwives and feldshers (paramedics focusing on internal medicine and some basic surgical skills). In general, midwives' skills need to be selectively upgraded in order to enable them to be of real assistance to patients and not only to assist the doctor—as is the case in many countries at present.

In upgrading equipment, primary care centers, too, should be reinforced at least to such an extent that high-risk pregnancies can be diagnosed and referred to the next level of health care in a timely manner. Primary health care centers also need to be able to deal with some obstetric emergencies and must have the appropriate essential drugs.

Antenatal care practices and policies need to be reviewed with respect to number of visits made and the type of examination to be performed at each visit. In obstetric practice, the broader concept of perinatal care for the health of the mother and the child should be widely introduced. Early breastfeeding (as recommended in the joint WHO–UNICEF statement on ten steps to successful breast feeding), rooming-in, and more active involvement of fathers in the perinatal period have been shown to contribute to a decrease in postnatal complications in both the mother and the infant.

Just like antenatal care, the concepts of postnatal care in the hospital and thereafter in the home should be reviewed. For instance, provision of community health workers who will help young mothers to cope with a newborn at home and follow-up on the health of the mother has been shown to be beneficial and cost-effective.

Finally, the prevention of cancer of the reproductive tract should be a regular component of primary health care. At present, screening programs are nonexistent or underdeveloped, which leads to the detection of cancers at a late stage, with a subsequently high cancer mortality, in particular from cervical cancer. Screening for cervical cancer could be integrated into polyclinics for women, as could breast cancer screening.

Conclusions

Reproductive ill health is a major public health concern in the countries of Central and Eastern Europe and the Newly Independent States. Only a strong commitment on the part of health policymakers, assistance and commitment from the international community, and a comprehensive interdisciplinary approach will significantly reduce present levels of morbidity and mortality in women and children in this subregion. The magnitude of the problem calls for urgent and radical action, and the World Health Organization remains ready to contribute through technical support, training, and research.

Bibliography

WHO Regional Office for Europe. 1995. *Highlights on women's health in Europe.* Doc: EUR/ICP/FMLY 94 01/PB02. Copenhagen: World Health Organization.

WHO 1995. *Maternal and infant health and family planning in the Central Asian Republics, Azerbaijan, and Kazakhstan (CARAK): proceedings of a meeting, Tashkent 1994.* Copenhagen: World Health Organization.

WHO 1995. *Women's health institutions; report on a WHO meeting, Vienna, Austria, 22–23 September 1995.* Copenhagen: World Health Organization.

WHO Regional Office for Europe and United Nations Population Fund. 1995. *Family planning and reproductive health in CCEE/NIS.* Copenhagen: World Health Organization.

WHO Regional Office for Europe. 1997. *Health for All database.*

WHO 1995. European Country Reports on Women's Health (unpublished).